Marie Weil
Editor

WITHDRAWN

Community Practice:
Models in Action

Pre-publication
REVIEWS,
COMMENTARIES,
EVALUATIONS . . .

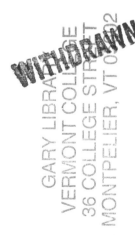

T his edited volume should be of
paramount interest to all would-
be community practice professionals.
Weil has compiled a text that seeks to
empower practitioners–primarily community organizers, social planners and
community developers–so that they are
best able to choose the most apposite
approach to unique community situations and problems. In my view the text
stands alone among macro texts in its
timeliness, comprehensiveness, and
contribution to strategy development.
The work could well become a classic in
that it not only emphasizes what practitioners need to know to be effective, but
also demonstrates how new theory
relates to current practice methods. This
is must reading for educators, students,
researchers and practitioners in the
community practice arena.

Moses Newsome, Jr., PhD
Dean, School of Social Work, Norfolk State
University, and President, Council on
Social Work Education

More pre-publication
REVIEWS, COMMENTARIES, EVALUATIONS . . .

I n *Community Practice: Models in Action* Marie Weil has presented a marvelous companion piece to her earlier edited volume, *Community Practice: Conceptual Models.*

Action places the theory in context. Specific examples give students and practitioners the authentic feel of CO practice, with its many organizations, competing interests, strains on the role of the worker, and fast pace of change. We see community-based development organizations interacting with banks. We see leadership development in context. CO has always had task goals and process goals and this collection reminds us all that what seems clear in the classroom is confounded and compounded in community.

John E. Tropman, PhD
School of Social Work, University of Michigan

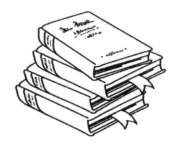

W eil's book offers several well-conceived models for community practice by leading authors in the field. These models are very relevant today when so much is changing in public and private sectors that affects community life and services. With reductions at the state and federal levels more is expected from the community, and these well-informed, thoughtful and insightful syntheses provide some avenues for effective community practice. Several also provide useful case examples to support their models. The book will be useful to community researchers and practitioners as well as to educators.

Rosemary C. Sarri
Professor Emerita, and Faculty Associate, Inst. for Social Research University of Michigan School of Social Work

More pre-publication
REVIEWS, COMMENTARIES, EVALUATIONS . . .

This well-written and idea-rich collection of articles explores the underdeveloped arena of community practice models placed into action. Neither too academically pedantic or prescriptive, nor limited and "cook-bookish," it moves effectively from considerations of model-building to applying model ideas in organizations and communities. It challenges the reader to consider a wide array of possible ideas and approaches from several community work perspectives; and an even wider array of perspective (e.g. feminist, multicultural, rural) are reflected and respected in this volume.

This volume succeeds in capturing the current thinking in the field of community work: a rich array of perspectives and approaches, grounded in both theory and practice. And it sets forth a wealth of ideas that students or community workers can use to define their own work. This is a fine book to wrestle with: it opens up practice possibilities without dictating why or how to think in using them. Readers should come away invigorated with the health of this field and the myriad practice possibilities open to them.

Scott Wilson
Co-author, Organizing for Power and Empowerment

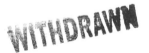

The Haworth Press, Inc.

Community Practice: Models in Action

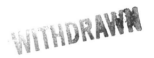

Community Practice: Models in Action

Marie Weil, DSW
Editor

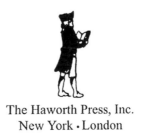

The Haworth Press, Inc.
New York • London

27.95

Community Practice: Models in Action has also been published as *Journal of Community Practice,* Volume 4, Number 1 1997.

Cover design by Donna M. Brooks

The Haworth Press, Inc., 10 Alice Street, Binghamton, NY 13904-1580 USA

Library of Congress Cataloging-in-Publication Data

Community practice : models in action / Marie Weil, editor.
     p. cm.
     "Also published as Journal of community practice, vol. 4, no. 1, 1997."
     Includes bibliographical references and index.
     ISBN 0-7890-0037-7 (alk. paper).–ISBN 0-7890-0046-6 (pbk.: alk. paper)
     1. Social service. 2. Community development. 3. Community organization. I. Weil, Marie, 1941- .
HV40.C6273 1997
361.8–dc21
                                           97-2327
                                           CIP

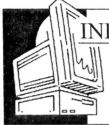

INDEXING & ABSTRACTING

Contributions to this publication are selectively indexed or abstracted in print, electronic, online, or CD-ROM version(s) of the reference tools and information services listed below. This list is current as of the copyright date of this publication. See the end of this section for additional notes.

- *Alternative Press Index,* Alternative Press Center, Inc., P.O. Box 33109, Baltimore, MD 21218-0401
- *Applied Social Sciences Index & Abstracts (ASSIA) (Online: ASSI via Data-Star) (CDRom: ASSIA Plus),* Bowker-Saur Limited, Maypole House, Maypole Road, East Grinstead, West Sussex RH19 1HH, England
- *caredata CD: the social and community care database,* National Institute for Social Work, 5 Tavistock Place, London WC1H 9SS, England
- *CINAHL (Cumulative Index to Nursing & Allied Health Literature, in print, also on CD-ROM from CD PLUS, EBSCO, and SilverPlatter, and online from CDP Online (formerly BRS), Data-Star, and PaperChase (Support materials include Subject Heading List, Database Search Guide, and instructional video),* CINAHL Information Systems, P.O. Box 871/1509 Wilson Terrace, Glendale, CA 91209-0871
- *CNPIEC Reference Guide: Chinese National Directory of Foreign Periodicals,* P.O. Box 88, Beijing, People's Republic of China
- *CPcurrents,* ITServices, 3301 Alta Arden #3, Sacramento, CA 95825
- *Economic Literature Index (Journal of Economic Literature) print version plus OnLine Abstracts (on Dialog) plus EconLit on CD-ROM (American Economic Association),* American Economic Association Publication, 4615 Fifth Avenue, Pittsburgh, PA 15213-3661
- *Family Studies Database (online and CD/ROM),* National Information Services Corporation, 306 East Baltimore Pike, 2nd Floor, Media, PA 19063

(continued)

- ***Family Violence & Sexual Assault Bulletin,*** Family Violence & Sexual Assault Institute, 1121 East South East Loop 323, Ste. 130, Tyler, TX 75701
- ***Guide to Social Science & Religion in Periodical Literature,*** National Periodical Library, P.O. Box 3278, Clearwater, FL 34630
- ***Human Resources Abstracts (HRA),*** Sage Publications, Inc., 2455 Teller Road, Newbury Park, CA 91320
- ***IBZ International Bibliography of Periodical Literature,*** Zeller Verlag GmbH & Co., P.O.B. 1949, d-49009 Osnabruck, Germany
- ***Index to Periodical Articles Related to Law,*** University of Texas, 727 East 26th Street, Austin, TX 78705
- ***International Political Science Abstracts,*** 27 Rue Saint-Guillaume, F-75337 Paris, Cedex 07, France
- ***INTERNET ACCESS (& additional networks) Bulletin Board for Libraries ("BUBL"), coverage of information resources on INTERNET, JANET, and other networks.***
  - JANET X. 29: UK.AC.BATH.BUBL or 00006012101300
  - TELNET: BUBL.BATH.AC.UK or 138.38.32.45 login 'bubl'
  - Gopher: BUBL.BATH.AC.UK (138.32.32.45). Port 7070
  - World Wide Web: http://www.bubl.bath.ac.uk./BUBL/home.html
  - NISSWAIS: telnetniss.ac.uk (for the NISS gateway)
  The Andersonian Library, Curran Building, 101 St. James Road, Glasgow G4 ONS, Scotland
- ***National Library Database on Homelessness,*** National Coalition for the Homeless, 1612 K Street, NW, #1004, Homelessness Information Exchange, Washington, DC 20006
- ***Operations Research/Management Science,*** Executive Sciences Institute, 1005 Mississippi Avenue, Davenport, IA 52803
- ***Public Affairs Information Bulletin (PAIS),*** Public Affairs Information Service, Inc., 521 West 43rd Street, New York, NY 10036-4396
- ***Rural Development Abstracts (CAB Abstracts), c/o CAB International/CAB ACCESS . . . available in print, diskettes updated weekly, and on INTERNET. Providing full bibliographic listings, author affiliation, augmented keyword searching,*** CAB International, P.O. Box 100, Wallingford Oxon OX10 8DE, United Kingdom

(continued)

- *Sage Family Studies Abstracts (SFSA),* Sage Publications, Inc., 2455 Teller Road, Newbury Park, CA 91320

- *Social Work Abstracts,* National Association of Social Workers, 750 First Street NW, 8th Floor, Washington, DC 20002

- *Sociological Abstracts (SA),* Sociological Abstracts, Inc., P.O. Box 22206, San Diego, CA 92192-0206

- *Transportation Research Abstracts,* National Research Council, 2101 Constitution Avenue NW, GR314, Washington, DC 20418

SPECIAL BIBLIOGRAPHIC NOTES

related to special journal issues (separates)
and indexing/abstracting

☐ indexing/abstracting services in this list will also cover material in any "separate" that is co-published simultaneously with Haworth's special thematic journal issue or DocuSerial. Indexing/abstracting usually covers material at the article/chapter level.

☐ monographic co-editions are intended for either non-subscribers or libraries which intend to purchase a second copy for their circulating collections.

☐ monographic co-editions are reported to all jobbers/wholesalers/approval plans. The source journal is listed as the "series" to assist the prevention of duplicate purchasing in the same manner utilized for books-in-series.

☐ to facilitate user/access services all indexing/abstracting services are encouraged to utilize the co-indexing entry note indicated at the bottom of the first page of each article/chapter/contribution.

☐ this is intended to assist a library user of any reference tool (whether print, electronic, online, or CD-ROM) to locate the monographic version if the library has purchased this version but not a subscription to the source journal.

☐ individual articles/chapters in any Haworth publication are also available through the Haworth Document Delivery Services (HDDS).

ABOUT THE EDITOR

Marie Weil, DSW, is Professor at the School of Social Work of the University of North Carolina at Chapel Hill where she serves as Director of the School's Community Social Work Program. Dr. Weil is first author of "Community Practice Models" and coauthor of "Citizen Participation" chapters in the 1995 Edition of the *Encyclopedia of Social Work*. Her recent publications include "Community Building: Building Community Practice" in *Social Work* and a forthcoming chapter, "Women, Community, and Development." She served as co-chair of the "Women, Community, and Sustainable Development" forum at UNC-CH in May 1996. She has been engaged in the development of the Association for Community Organization and Social Administration (ACOSA) from its inception. She is currently engaged in research on grassroots organizations and the nonprofit sector.

Community Practice: Models in Action

CONTENTS

Introduction: Models of Community Practice in Action   1
     Marie Weil, DSW

Core Concepts for Community Change   11
     Barry Checkoway, PhD

Public Life in Gulfton: Multiple Publics and Models
     of Community Organization   31
     Lisa Taaffe, LMSW
     Robert Fisher, PhD

Being a Conscience and a Carpenter: Interpretations
     of the Community-Based Development Model   57
     Herbert J. Rubin, PhD

Conceptual Framework of Coalitions
     in an Organizational Context   91
     Maria Roberts-DeGennaro, PhD

Leadership: Realizing Concepts Through Creative Process   109
     Si Kahn, PhD

Index   137

Introduction:
Models of Community Practice in Action

Marie Weil, DSW

Conceptual models for community work are schemas that shape and define an approach to practice. Models knit together theoretical concepts and connect them to guidelines for action; and as such, serve as powerful teaching, planning, analytic, and self-evaluation tools for community practice. Models for practice should distinguish among purposes, methods, activities, and roles to assist practitioners in selecting the most appropriate approach to a particular community or situation at a particular time.

Ann Jeffries argues that models of practice seek to specify a basic orientation to practice and clarify "the strategies, roles and skills that are likely to be most useful given the particular approach chosen" (1996, p. 102). Her definition is useful in understanding both purpose and application:

> a model is a simplification of reality that is intended to order and clarify our perception of that reality while still encapsulating its essential characteristics. To have analytical value a model should specify key variables to be considered in assessing a situation in order to develop and evaluate possible action plans. Thus a model should enable prediction of likely outcomes if a particular plan of action is pursued. (Jeffries, 1996, p. 101)

[Haworth co-indexing entry note]: "Introduction: Models of Community Practice in Action." Weil, Marie. Co-published simultaneously in *Journal of Community Practice* (The Haworth Press, Inc.) Vol. 4, No. 1, 1997, pp. 1-9; and: *Community Practice: Models in Action* (ed: Marie Weil) The Haworth Press, Inc., 1997, pp. 1-9. Single or multiple copies of this article are available for a fee from The Haworth Document Delivery Service [1-800-342-9678, 9:00 a.m. - 5:00 p.m. (EST). E-mail address: getinfo@ haworth.com].

Jeffries' definition is especially useful in its reminder that a model must necessarily be a "simplification" or abstraction of reality. Typologies of models are grounded in two arenas: (a) in-depth examination of varieties of practice experience, that is investigation of variation within particular models; and (b) analytical work to examine commonalities and distinguishing characteristics among diverse models. Comparable factors are abstracted from multiple examples to provide a simplified representation of commonalities. From these examples, a general description that specifies the basic approach and salient characteristics of an intervention model can be used to guide actions in new practice situations. Models are, therefore, built on and abstracted from practice realities (Gamble, 1996). In the application of a model to a specific community, situation, or issue, it is critical to carefully analyze the particular action group (or groups) and the salient issues related to desired outcomes (Weil & Gamble, 1995). A second critical step in applying a model to a specific situation is to analyze the particular context–including economic/political/social forces and race/ethnicity/gender issues (Gamble, 1996). These analyses should be combined to focus on the goals and intended outcomes for action.

Practice models typically use concepts to formulate and synthesize complex ideas. Some models are purely conceptual, in that they focus on abstracting complex social realities and explaining behavior. Concepts are the building blocks for models and theories. A concept is an idea–an understanding of a phenomenon or experience: *liberty* is a concept, *community* is a concept as are *system* and *ecology*. A purely conceptual model of a theory illustrates, explains, or predicts behavior or social phenomena, while conceptual models of practice have a distinct purpose and go several steps further. Practice models use concepts and explanation not just to understand and/or predict social phenomena, but most centrally to guide action and intervention toward chosen goals.

Practice models typically specify comparative characteristics such as (a) those related to goals and desired outcomes, change target, constituency, scope of concern, and workers' roles (Weil & Gamble, 1995); (b) Rothman's twelve major practice variables (1979; 1970); (c) Popple's focus on comparing and contrasting strategies, worker's primary roles, practice examples and key texts

(1996); or (d) Hyde's focus on types of community interventions, organizational types and feminist examples (1996). Each of these model typologies seeks to guide thinking and provide the basis for strategy development. While models are often depicted in "boxes" to display the typology and contrast approaches, they should serve as analytical tools and not be viewed as rigid prescriptions. Models, that is, should be used to structure thinking and provide a basis for creative choices and action in practice.

The reality that models of community practice are not "pure" or totally differentiated has been long recognized. In 1979, Rothman adapted his initial article to discuss the "mixing and phasing" of models in actual practice; and his most recent revision elaborates that process (Rothman, 1979, 1996). In Rothman's new revision of his typology, he amply illustrates that models can not only be mixed and phased, but that hybrid "mixed models" such as action/planning or planning/development are prevalent in practice (Rothman, 1996). When hybrid models are used or when strategies are mixed and/or phased, it remains important to know which strategies/models are being used toward which goals and what overall mission encompasses and guides the use of multiple models.

In practice, models may succeed each other as in a move from organizing to local social planning and service development (Mondros & Wilson, 1994); or different programs of a community-based organization might use distinct models in different components of its work. For example, an organization whose basic mission is economic development might in response to particular community contexts also decide to plan and implement specific social services such as eldercare or child daycare. In these instances, such services are an investment in the community and may support or connect to other economic and community development efforts (NCCED, 1990).

As used here, a model is not intended to signify an isolated or fixed approach with impermeable boundaries. Given the needs of particular situations, models will be mixed and phased to be most effective in the current situation and stage of organizational or community development. Creativity and adaptability arise from the process of mixing and phasing; however, it is very useful to have a primary model in mind—so participants can know what is being mixed and/or phased—and so that theory and knowledge, research concepts and findings can be used to strengthen and refine practice interventions.

The application of a conceptual model can move practice activities beyond a reactive stance to a proactive, planned, and strategic intervention. In any community practice project, one of the chief responsibilities of the worker is to assist in assessing and selecting appropriate and useful models for guiding choices and activities. In addition to providing a framework for analyzing current purposes, goals, strategies and tactics, well-developed practice models will incorporate a value analysis to use in selecting strategies. In given situations, workers may (1) apply a known practice model with its related theories, concepts, knowledge, and values, (2) adapt or combine concepts and models for the current situation, or (3) construct a conceptual model selecting appropriate theories, research, and values to analyze and plan actions for a particular situation. Conceptual models are a major means of translating theory and ideas into strategies for action and methods of intervention. Models therefore are critical tools to frame thinking and action.

In an article in the 19th Edition of the *Encyclopedia of Social Work*, Weil and Gamble argue that current models of community practice have evolved from the earliest traditions in community practice: the Settlement movement, the Charity Organization Society movement, and the Rural Development movement (Weil & Gamble, 1995). The Labor movement and the organizing and development histories of ethnic and racial groups likewise have made major contributions to the development of community practice models (Betten & Austin, 1990; Rivera & Erlich, 1992). While considerable work remains to refine and interpret the theoretical base of each of the current models, their evolution is important in understanding community practice and clarifying the commonalities and differences among practice approaches.

In the companion volume to this work, *Community Practice: Conceptual Models* (1996), a variety of conceptual and practice model approaches are presented: Rothman's interweaving of community intervention approaches; Jeffries' analytic framework; Hyde's feminist analysis and application across Rothman's typology; and Popple's presentation of current models in the United Kingdom; as well as an example of use of ecological theory to guide community practice (MacNair) and an historical perspective on community practice model development (Weil). That set of chapters presents the state of the art in community practice typologies.

This volume presents examples of three of the basic community practice models in action—that is, in-depth analyses of current issues and examples of: community organization, community economic development, and coalition building. It begins with a chapter analyzing the core concepts applicable in all community change processes and concludes with a chapter that illustrates the engagement of creativity and affirmation in leadership development processes. This second volume therefore builds on and informs the more abstract and general presentation of typologies and frameworks in the first volume. As noted in the introduction to the companion volume, theory and models should be tested and examined in relation to changing contexts, shifting social forces, and new realities. The chapters in this volume reground and test models through detailed examinations of current practice experiences. They bring new theory to bear in analysis of current practice, examine changes, and document new or hybrid emphases in basic models.

Barry Checkoway presents and analyzes core concepts and praxis principles that relate to all major models of intervention for community change. Change processes are taken as the central factor in community-based intervention. He has derived these concepts/ principles from research in social work, public health, urban planning, and related fields and from practice descriptions of community organization, social planning, and neighborhood development. His presentation is enriched by comparisons of rural with urban contexts and post industrial-societies with developing areas in various parts of the world. The chapter is useful in its presentation of change as a process that can be shaped to strengthen community. Change processes are used to illustrate the combining of strategies and skills. Readers are encouraged to test out the concepts and principles discussed and adapt them or develop their own core concepts to guide work directed toward planned community change. The chapter provides perspective on the central importance of clear concepts and principles to guide practice.

In "Public Life in Gulfton: Multiple Publics and Models of Community Organization," Lisa Taaffe and Robert Fisher explain the meaning and importance of the concepts of *public life* and *multiple publics*. They examine the current political, policy, and practice shifts related to the role of the public sector and the phenomena of increasing privatization and analyze these shifts in relation to the construction of civil society. They stress the impact of the post-industrial global economy on communities. After documenting their research on six community organizations in Gulfton, they analyze the complexity of life in current heterogeneous urban neighborhoods, concluding that the often fractious relations among such groups with diverse interests and aims illustrate a shift toward "organizing based on communities of interest–racial/ethnic/political–as well as communities of place." While relations among such groups may be contentious, in a society of increasing privatization, these diverse and polyvocal community organizations they hold, "serve a critical secondary role of maintaining and invigorating public life." Applying a postmodern perspective, they argue that these diverse and competing groups "may contribute to the larger social change project of rebuilding public and community life around the ideals of democratic process, cultural diversity, and social struggle."

In "Being a Conscience and a Carpenter: Interpretations of the Community-Based Development Model," Herbert J. Rubin argues in contrast to considerable literature that Community-Based Development Organizations (CBDOs) successfully link development activities with advocacy and services. In a three-year project, Rubin conducted research on models and practices of exemplary CBDOs and here describes central elements of a model for empowered community-based development. Leaders of sixty CBDOs were interviewed as well as activists from organizations that assist community developers. Quotes and examples from development activists illustrate their clear connections of advocacy and services to development projects as well as their constant struggle with the "double bottom line"–need for financial accountability and for adherence to the nonprofits' social goals. Some respondents described an holistic model of community renewal and processes of coalition building that can create resources and an empowered community. Rubin's paper documents that concepts related to development have quite grounded meanings. He provides examples of organic theory formulated as those working on positive social change reflect on and interpret their experiences and actions. The article is a strong example of the use of research in model analysis and development. Rubin encourages learning from the activists interviewed and the thoughtful integration of development, activist, and social service strategies to rebuild and restore communities.

Maria Roberts-DeGennaro contributes a "Conceptual Framework of Coalitions in an Organizational Context." The chapter describes the roles coalitions can play in changing their sociopolitical contexts. She uses the political-economy perspective to define coalition building and elaborates five coalition models distinguished by purpose. Case examples illustrate practice applications and major functions of the five coalition models focused on: information and resource sharing; technical assistance; self-regulating; planning and coordination; and advocacy. Practice considerations are analyzed with an emphasis on coalitions convening for sociopolitical action in response to shifts in the political-economic environment. Through its examination of the various roles that coalitions take for social action, the article builds the knowledge base and provides ideas useful for further theory development about the nature and purposes of coalitions, and about function-related behaviors and strategies in coalition building.

Each of the three models in action presented in this volume, community organizing, community economic development, and coalition building, are anchored in the history of community practice. However, for a model to have relevance, it must be examined, analyzed, researched, and updated–tested in and against the realities of current practice and updated in relation to changing, economic, technological, social, political, and environmental conditions. In order for a model to be useful for teaching new practitioners and assisting local leaders in analyzing and developing strategies for local situations, it must be current, grounded in contemporary context, and provide exemplars for practice from which others can learn and adapt to comparable situations. The chapters included in this volume provide evidence of the value in using research to examine, develop, and update models.

In the concluding piece for this volume, Si Kahn, who as director of Grassroots Leadership has done extensive training for leadership, as well as direct organizing, illustrates the use of an interactive process to tap into the creativity of participants. The article provides a brief history, context, and theory for community organizing, drawing from concepts of culture, community, and power. It illustrates a leadership development experience that provides affirmation and inspiration for the tough work of organizing. The process validates participatory leadership, verbally and visually illustrates strengths of participants, and liberates energy for that work. All too often, creativity is not recognized or acknowledged for the central part of organizing and development work that it is. Analytic processes are weakened if they are not combined with creative responses. The "I Am a Leader Because" exercise as Kahn describes it is not just an icebreaker in leadership development, but a powerful instrument of communication, celebration, affirmation, and creation of shared meaning. It cuts through the purely mental processes and reaches the deeper sense of commitment that draws people into organizing and development work.

Commitment is an essential ingredient for community workers and community leaders–and commitment needs to be nurtured and refueled. Leaders need opportunities to reflect and regenerate; community workers also need that process, and in addition need to know how to facilitate the process to help individuals and groups grow and develop toward their goals. Creativity is a large part of the art of practice and needs further examination as well as nurture and expansion.

In combination, these chapters give guidance for work, research, and further exploration in major areas of community practice. They strengthen conceptualizations and provide means for serious examination of current realities of practice. They raise questions about traditional models and identify changing contextual and environmental issues that must be taken into account and analyzed in order to adapt practice and models to current realities. They provide opportunities to engage creativity in leadership development and strategy selection. Most importantly, perhaps, they raise questions for ongoing model development and applications that can help to guide research and theory building and foster creativity in practice.

REFERENCES

Betten, N. & Austin, M. J. (Eds.) (1990). *The roots of community organizing, 1917-1939*. Philadelphia: Temple University Press.

Gamble, D. (September 1, 1997). Personal communication.

Hyde, C. (1996). A feminist response to Rothman's "Interweaving of community intervention approaches" in M. Weil (Ed.), *Journal of Community Practice*, 3(3/4), pp. 127-145.

Jeffries, A. (1996). Modeling community work: An analytical framework for practice, in M. Weil (Ed.), *Journal of Community Practice*, 3(3/4), pp. 101-125.

MacHair, R. H. (1996). Theory for community practice in social work: The example of ecological community practice, in M. Weil (Ed.), *Journal of Community Practice*, 3(3/4), pp. 181-202.

Mondros, J. B. & Wilson, S. M. (1994). *Organizing for Power and Empowerment.* New York: Columbia University Press.

National Congress for Community Economic Development. (November, 1990). *Human investment: Community profits. Social Services and Economic Development Task Force: Report and Recommendations.* Washington DC: NCCED.

Popple, K. (1996). Community work: British models, in M. Weil (Ed.), *Journal of Community Practice*, 3(3/4), pp. 147-179.

Rivera F. G. & Erlich, J. L. (Eds.) (1992). *Community organizing in a diverse society.* Boston: Allyn and Bacon.

Rothman, J. (1996). The interweaving of community intervention approaches, in M. Weil (Ed.), *Journal of Community Practice*, 3(3/4), pp. 69-99.

Rothman, J. (1979). Three models of community organization practice, their mixing and phasing. In F. Cox, J. Erlich, J. Rothman, & J. Tropman (Eds.), *Strategies of community organization* pp. 25-44. Itasca, IL: Peacock Publishers.

Rothman, J. (1970). Three models of community organization, in F. Cox, J. Erlich, J. Rothman, and J. Tropman (Eds.), *Strategies of community organization.* Itasca, IL: Peacock Publishers.

Weil, M. (Ed.) (1996). *Community Practice: Conceptual Models.* New York: The Haworth Press, Inc., co-published as *Journal of Community Practice*, 3(3/4).

Weil, M. (1996). Introduction in M. Weil (Ed.), *Journal of Community Practice*, 3(3/4), pp. 1-3.

Weil, M. (1996). Model development in community practice: An historical perspective, in M. Weil (Ed.), *Journal of Community Practice*, 3(3/4), pp. 5-67.

Weil, M. & Gamble, D. (1995). Community practice models, in R. L. Edwards, (Ed.). *Encyclopedia of social work, Nineteenth Edition.* Washington, DC: NASW.

Core Concepts for Community Change

Barry Checkoway, PhD

SUMMARY. This paper presents several core concepts or praxis principles for creating community change. It provides perspectives on change as a process of strengthening community and joining together through several strategies and skills. It draws upon research in social work, urban planning, public health, and related fields; on practice in community organization, social planning, and neighborhood development; and on work with rural and urban communities in industrial countries and developing areas worldwide. It concludes by challenging the reader to develop his or her own core concepts for community change. *[Article copies available for a fee from The Haworth Document Delivery Service: 1-800-342-9678. E-mail address: getinfo@haworth.com]*

KEYWORDS. Community change, community development, multicultural organizing, empowerment

Core concepts are abstract ideas generalized from particular situations. They reduce such situations to their fundamentals, expressing their basic elements in a few summary words. When used in reference to fields like community change, they take on some of the qualities of "praxis principles" with potential to integrate information about "thought" and "action" in a new combination.

Barry Checkoway is Professor of Social Work and Urban Planning at the University of Michigan.

Address correspondence to: Barry Checkoway, School of Social Work, University of Michigan, Ann Arbor, MI 48109.

[Haworth co-indexing entry note]: "Core Concepts for Community Change." Checkoway, Barry. Co-published simultaneously in *Journal of Community Practice* (The Haworth Press, Inc.) Vol. 4, No. 1, 1997, pp. 11-29; and: *Community Practice: Models in Action* (ed: Marie Weil) The Haworth Press, Inc., 1997, pp. 11-29. Single or multiple copies of this article are available for a fee from The Haworth Document Delivery Service [1-800-342-9678, 9:00 a.m. - 5:00 p.m. (EST). E-mail address: getinfo@ haworth.com].

Core concepts can serve positive purposes for community change. First, they can form the basis for decisions about actions to take in the community. When people are faced with a decision among various possibilities, for example, core concepts can provide a reminder of purpose or an expression of vision that helps clarify the choice.

Second, they can cause an awakening that is truly transformational. Amidst the routine confusion of everyday events, people suddenly put the pieces together and make sense of their situation in a new way. When people "see" an underlying concept that sheds new light on their lives, it can "change their world" and motivate them to pursue new forms of social action. In some cases, this awakening can be revolutionary (Fanon, 1968; Freire, 1970; Gatt-Fly, 1983).

Where do core concepts come from? Ideally, people establish their own principles through a process in which they themselves participate. Instead, however, many principles come as traditions from the past, tenets from ideological movements, or commands from beneficent or repressive regimes. Such concepts may have power behind them, but their authority is always arguable when they do not derive from the people themselves.

Educators and trainers often communicate core concepts as a form of "do this!" knowledge with or without having a scientific basis for their statements. Some people are eager to have this type of expert information, but the potential for empowerment is greater when people think for themselves rather than depend upon professionals. This contrasts with the pattern in which professionals expropriate knowledge and treat people like passive recipients of services rather than as active participants in the process. When practice wisdom derives from collective reflection, it reappropriates knowledge and promotes participation in the community (Brown, 1993; Gaventa, 1988).

This article is intended for people who have potential to create community change, and for those who might help others learn more about the process. It assumes that these people are limitless in numbers and boundless in opportunities–including ordinary citizens and local leaders, professional practitioners and change-agents, and teachers and trainers in schools and communities. It recognizes that people will differ in their roles, but that all will benefit from reflecting upon experience and learning lessons for future action. It offers some core concepts based on research and practice, but does not prescribe them as the only ones, and challenges you to formulate your own.

Following are some core concepts for community change. They are based on my knowledge of practice theory and process models in social work, urban planning, and related fields; on empirical research on practice initiatives in community organization, social planning, and neighborhood development; and on practice in rural and urban communities in industrial countries and developing areas worldwide. My knowledge base has led me to these particular concepts, but different ways of knowing should surely produce different areas. If you question these concepts, and substitute your own, my purpose will be served.

It would be possible for some people to search for and find an overall pattern or model in this presentation of concepts. For example, some concepts focus on community and organization as forms of intervention, others on the types of people and strategies involved in the process, and others on believing in change and its cultural context. I appreciate the need to find an overall pattern, but do not want to suggest that there is single sequencing of elements to be followed. On the contrary, I believe that there is no single model that fits all approaches to practice, and, again, that the key is to formulate your own concepts and to create a framework that fits your particular situation.

STRENGTHENING COMMUNITY

Community is a process of people acting collectively with others who share some common concern. This is not the only meaning of the term, which also refers to a place where people live, or a group of people with similar interests, or relationships which have social cohesion or continuity in time. These other meanings may find expression in the process, but they are not the process itself (Checkoway, 1991; Suttles, 1972).

Strengthening community can take various forms, such as organizing a group for social action, planning a local program, or developing a neighborhood service. As long as people are acting collectively, then the process is taking place. Used this way, community is more than a noun or adjective, but also a verb that refers to the process as well as its product. Perhaps a better term for the process is not community, but "community-building."

Community is one of several levels of intervention in society. For example, there are personal or interpersonal interventions with individuals and families; organizational approaches to leadership and management of institutions; and macroscale efforts to influence public policy in the larger society. Community interventions are the ones that take collective action and mediate between the individual and the society. Community is an important level of intervention, but it is not the only one.

Community-building is facilitated or limited by the unit that is selected for change (Eng, 1988). Emphasis is often placed on the community as a spatial unit or physical place—such as a village or a neighborhood—whose boundaries facilitate or limit the organizing process (Unger & Wandersman, 1985). Some analysts argue that place is being replaced by "community without propinquity," facilitated by transportation or telecommunications technology enabling some people to join together in nonspatial ways (Catalfo, 1993; Webber, 1963). Nonspatial community is contingent upon access to technology, whereas place remains important to those whose resources are limited.

Some people care about the "general welfare" of the "community as a whole." Looking down from the municipal building, for example, they identify issues whose resolution will presumably benefit the whole community. However, most communities are not monolithic; they include various groups whose differences call for more multicultural forms of intervention. People who care about the whole community often care about no one community and benefit some segments more than others (Rivera & Erlich, 1992; Heskin & Heffner, 1987).

Community-building also has limitations as a form of intervention. First, there are personal crises that require immediate action by an experienced professional. It is as inappropriate for individuals to take some of their personal troubles to a community meeting, as it is for community groups to seek solace for neighborhood problems in the office of a psychotherapist. Second, communities vary in their levels of readiness for change. Some "healthy" or "competent" communities create change with fervor, whereas others lack resources or are unsure how to proceed (Cottrell, 1983; Iscoe, 1974; Lackey, 1987). Third, even the healthiest communities may have difficulties influencing the larger society in which they operate. Local communities should not be expected to solve problems whose causes lie elsewhere, or whose solutions are beyond their reach.

However, the forces which limit community-building do not diminish its significance as a "unit of solution" in the world (Steuart, 1993). Indeed, obstacles are a normal part of the change process, and successful efforts to overcome them amplify the potential of community-building as a form of intervention. What is *your* community? What is your *unit* of solution?

JOINING TOGETHER, IN SOLIDARITY

Imagine a series of "stick figure" drawings moving across a piece of paper. First there is a person standing alone, then the person is talking with two others, and then the three are bringing a group together in front of a hut in the village. Suddenly the whole group comes to life. They are alive with emotion, everyone wanting to speak in animated fashion. There is energy that could lead to a new level of collective action. It is like a fire whose combined ingredients give light and warmth; the fire starts with a single match, and burns because the twigs catch alight and the logs fuel the flame (Hope & Timmel, 1984).

The concept is that a number of people joining together in solidarity can accomplish more than one person acting alone. It is the notion of "collective action," "strength in unity," or the Swahili term *Harambee,* "joining together."

Joining together helps people to realize that their individual problems have social causes and collective solutions. As individuals unite in solidarity, they reduce their isolation and interact with others in ways that have psychosocial benefits and contribute to their perceived and real power (Bandura, 1982; Checkoway, Freeman, & Hovaguimian, 1988). This does not devalue the importance of individual initiative, but instead recognizes the strength that comes from joining together.

Solidarity can build upon common concerns that arise from a place in which people live or work, or from preexisting social or cultural characteristics such as race or gender. These characteristics have potential for solidarity, but are insufficient to build community in the absence of joining together. People who share common concerns still need some sort of process to make them salient for the purpose of community-building.

GETTING ORGANIZED

Community change can start with unplanned actions or random events, but it is only when people get organized that lasting change takes place.

"Getting organized" is the process by which people develop some sort of structure for joining together over time. It takes its most basic expression when individuals form into a coherent unity and establish a mechanism for systematic planning and limited effort. This "organizing moment" is a key dynamic in the process of community change (Biddle & Biddle, 1965).

"Organizing" is the process by which individuals work together to accomplish more than any one of them acting alone (Kahn, 1991; Kendall, 1991; Rubin & Rubin, 1992; Staples, 1984). It is illustrated by an image of individuals isolated together in a row of small cramped cells, then pushing against the walls that separate them, then breaking through the walls and touching others, and finally standing strong with their arms linked together in a single unit (Speeter, 1978). This process transcends time and place, and finds its expression in sayings worldwide, such as in Mauritania: "Two eyes see better than one" or Madagascar: "Cross the river in a crowd, and the crocodile won't eat you" or Ethiopia: "When spider webs unite, they can tie up the lion" (Hope & Timmel, 1984).

Organizing is an empowering process that enhances psychosocial well-being. It enables individuals to increase their individual coping capacity, personal confidence, and feelings of control. Its therapeutic effects are especially important for individuals whose alienation keeps them from organizing on their own behalf, or whose displacement causes them to "blame themselves" for the forces acting upon them (Minkler, 1990; Rappaport, 1981; Ryun, 1976; Zimmerman, 1992).

Organizing builds collective capacity and a "sense of community." Strategy can include stages in which people form groups to win victories on initial issues that enable them to strengthen their structural organization and to take on more major issues. In one community, people organize to halt an expressway from encroaching on their area, form an areawide coalition of organizations, and plan programs of their own. In another community, they organize to protest slum landlords, rehabilitate abandoned housing, and develop services responsive to local needs. Sense of community is a catalyst for participation (Chavis & Wandersman, 1990; McMillan & Chavis, 1986).

"Organization" is the structure established for organizing over the long haul. It may include forms of problem-solving and program-planning, goal-setting and decision-making, role-definition and team-building, administrative structuring and organizational development. It may be informal or formal, collectivist or bureaucratic, and horizontal or vertical, depending upon the situation.

What is the appropriate organizational form for community change? Will it differ among rich and poor, Black and White, men and women? There is no single answer to these questions, except that good practice fits the appropriate form to the particular situation.

STARTING WITH PEOPLE

A central tenet of community change is that it should start with people who have concerns and who know what they want to accomplish. The premise is that people are the best judge of their own situation, and that the process should originate in the experience of the people themselves (Tweeten & Brinkman, 1976).

As part of their training, professionals learn how to assess the needs of their clients. For example, social workers take courses that teach techniques in how to approach their target populations, conduct interviews and ask questions about their lives, and gather information for diagnosis and intervention. The belief is that accurate information on client needs will make professionals more responsive to the people they serve.

However, needs assessment by providers for the purpose of service delivery is different from participatory assessment for the purpose of community change. Many methods of assessment are available, only some of which actively involve the community in the process. These methods take time and lack the status of those that treat respondents like human subjects–but they do start with the people themselves (Eng & Blanchard, 1991; Marti-Costa & Serrano-Garcia, 1987).

Also, the usual focus on the needs of people carries the risk of ignoring their substantial strengths, and making them dependent upon the professionals who assess and define their capacity. Endless emphasis on the deficits of people may result in losses of self-esteem or "learned helplessness" in which individuals feel unable to do things that otherwise are within their grasp (Garber & Seligman, 1980). It is especially important to appreciate the strengths of communities whose overemphasis on their disadvantages can cause them to lose confidence in themselves (McKnight & Kretzman, n.d.).

Are people the best judge of their own situation? Werner and Bower (1983) draw two pictures, one of an expert standing over a respondent and asking preconceived questions listed on a clipboard, the other of villagers sitting together and discussing their common interests with the help of an indigenous facilitator from the village. The caption reads: "For local health workers and their communities, the need is not to gather information. . . . but to gather everyone together and look at what they already know" (p. 6).

Do people know what they want and what is best for themselves, including their actual needs and potential strengths? Democratic ideology says that the people are sovereign in this type of knowledge. But if consciousness is a social construction that results from the form of a given society–and if people's expressed beliefs are not always of their own making–then what? Or if people have consciousness that may be viewed as harmful to them–such as the villagers who believe that their children's worms are caused by angry gods rather than by bacteria in the water, or the residents who attribute neighborhood decline to their own cultural flaws rather than to disinvestment by the banks–then what?

DEVELOPING LEADERSHIP

Who *are* the people? Are they the ordinary citizens, as in the Aristotelian sense that "the people at large should be sovereign rather than the few best"? This view gives primacy to the role of the average person, assumes that they are–or are becoming more–equal in their participation, and looks to the grassroots as the foundation for change (Kasperson & Breitbart, 1974).

Or are they the community leaders, such as the elected members of the town council or the officers of the neighborhood association? The politics of leadership is an admission of inequality rather than a reaffirmation of full participation, but it recognizes the role of representation, and is the prevalent form of democracy in the world today. Real leaders are indigenous and accountable representatives of the people whom they serve rather than the ones who are assigned to them from the outside (Pitkin, 1969).

Where are the leaders of the community? They are found by their formal positions in established institutions, although formal leaders are not always the real ones; by their reputations in getting things done, although perceptions of leadership are subject to change; by their influence in important decisions, although each decision may have its own patterns of influence; or by the scope of their participation, although the extent of participation is not necessarily a measure of its impact. It is possible to find them among the poorest people in the world, although this infrastructure is not readily accessible to outsiders (Tait & Bokenheimer, n.d.; Werner, 1993; Werner & Bower, 1983).

Which types of leaders are best? Should the leader be "authoritarian" by making a decision and announcing it to the community; or "consultative" by identifying the alternatives and asking the community for its input; or "enabling" by helping the community to identify its issues and facilitating its decisions? Again, the answers will vary with the situation (Hope & Timmel, 1984).

How can a community develop new leaders? This question is so fundamental that most communities tend to ignore it. Instead, they tend to appropriate leadership by promoting people who already hold positions in established institutions and who, as a result, are either unrepresentative of the community or unable to invest time for the job. However, community change offers opportunities to develop new leaders rather than to appropriate old ones–to identify people with potential and encourage them to lead (Checkoway, 1981).

AGENTS OF CHANGE

Community change has a history of voluntary action that arises from "the hearts and minds of the people," including indigenous individuals who emerge spontaneously and facilitate the process through their commitment to social values rather than through the promise of remuneration. Most of the world's great change-agents– such as Jesus Christ or Mahatma Gandhi–have been volunteers.

Recent years have witnessed an increase in the number of people with professional careers as agents of community change. This role is emerging in different ways in different areas–for example, promotura de salud, community organizer, adult educator, cultural worker, social animator–that together recognize some of the professional expertise and technical skills that are needed. In one or another area these individuals can create community change. They can enter a community, bring people together, and build a powerful organization. They can formulate an action strategy, build support for implementation, and generate one project from another.

There also are support networks that strengthen the work of change-agents. These networks include institutions with funding for proposals, communications vehicles to facilitate information exchange, interorganizational coalitions to develop alliances, and training programs to build community capacity. These networks are instrumental in the "resource mobilization" of some agents of change (Berger & Neuhaus, 1977; McCarthy & Zald, 1973).

One legacy of Saul Alinsky (1969, 1971) was to promote the role of the community organizer as a professional worker. According to Alinsky, community organization took trained workers with technical expertise and special skills. He distinguished among the "organizer," "leader," and "people," and sought to strengthen their collaboration. Professional expertise is no substitute for voluntary action, to be sure, but change-agents can contribute to the process (Horwitt, 1989; Reitzes & Reitzes, 1980).

SEVERAL STRATEGIES

There are several strategies, skills, and styles of community change. "Strategies" include approaches to mobilize individuals around issues through highly visible demonstrations, or to organize grass-roots groups for social action. They can involve people in policy planning through committees and meetings of government agencies, or advocate for groups by representing them in legislative or other established institutional arenas. They can raise critical consciousness through small group discussions, or develop neighborhood services of their own. These strategies are separable, each with its own empirical basis and practice pattern, but also with mixing and phasing among them (Checkoway, 1991; Rothman & Tropman, 1987).

"Skills" include practical tools to enter the community, assess local conditions, and formulate plans for program implementation. They include efforts to make contact with people, bring them together, and form and build organizations. They include efforts to identify and negotiate with decision makers, relate to other groups in the community, and develop the confidence and competence needed to keep the process going. There are various process models in community work which describe types of basic skills (Henderson & Thomas, 1987).

"Styles" affect the manner in which strategies and skills will be received or supported by the community. Conflict style assumes that power is scarce and that confrontation may be necessary for its redistribution; campaign style assumes that it is possible to persuade people to see things in a particular way; and consensus style assumes that power is abundant and that people are in relative agreement on how to share it (Warren, 1972). The selection of a style that fits in the community is sometimes more important than the issues themselves. People who are conflictual or consensual may avoid taking action on an important issue if the tactics are inappropriate to their style.

Strategic choice is a key diagnostic step in various fields of practice. For example, a teacher listens to the classroom discussion and asks an awakening question; a chess player conceptualizes the board and makes a move; and an athlete senses the action on the playing field and finds an opening. Just as these people diagnose their situation and take appropriate action, so too does an agent of community change. And some do it with more or less skill than others (Schon, 1983).

Like other fields, community change also has people who misdiagnose their situation and prescribe inappropriate action. For example, they are the ones who convince villagers to pray for forgiveness from the gods when the real cause of problems is the urbanization of the society; or who convince residents of their responsibility to sweep the streets when the real cause of litter is neglect by the sanitation department. Misdiagnosis can have harmful effects in any practice field.

Selecting an appropriate strategy, skill, or style is central to community change. Some people do it naturally, others learn by trial and error, and others ignore it altogether, although these last are ignorant indeed.

BELIEVING IN CHANGE

Basic to the process of creating change is a belief in its possibility. This belief is instrumental to the process, and also is an end in itself.

Believing in change has an uneven distribution, which Werner and Bower (1983) view as levels on a continuum. At one level are people who strongly believe that change is possible. They perceive that community problems have solutions over which they have control, they show confidence in their own ability, and they take decisive actions that produce results. These people are relatively few in number and tend to have disproportionate power.

At another level are people who are weaker in their orientation to change. They are aware of community problems, but only periodically try to do something about them. They participate in the community to a limited extent, but this is only occasional in occurrence. They are many in number and sometimes susceptible to mobilization. When this happens, it can be revolutionary, but it does not happen very often.

At another level are people who do not believe that change is possible. They face problems in their personal lives, but generally do not view them as issues around which to organize. They have informal support from family and friends, but often feel alienated from formal participation in the community. They appear to lack the consciousness needed to create change, although appearances can be deceiving and awakenings can occur when conditions are right.

What explains the differences in beliefs among people? Some analysts attribute them to characteristics of the people themselves, praising or blaming them for their own orientation. Others attribute them to the uneven distribution of resources that permits some people to organize more powerfully than others. Yet others attribute them to institutional patterns of privilege and oppression that discriminate among groups and shape their consciousness, which is not independent but instead results from these patterns. It is tragic when institutions rob people of their spirit and cause them to blame themselves for situations which are not of their making, but this "false consciousness" is a powerful force in the world (Hyde, 1994).

How can people help others to strengthen their own belief in the possibility of change? Freire (1970) describes a pedagogy in which individuals discuss the root causes of problems and strengthen their capacity for concerted action; Werner and Bower (1983) describe a process in which the facilitator asks "but why?" questions about the chain of causes and about the specific steps needed to alter the situation; and Horton (1990) discusses a school whose workshops draw people together to identify individual problems and develop collective solutions. For them, community change is an awakening process that motivates people for action (Hope & Timmel, 1984).

AN EMPOWERING PROCESS

Empowerment is a multilevel process by which people perceive that they have control over their situation. It can refer to an individual who feels a sense of personal control over his or her life; an organization that engages its members and influences the community of which it is a part; or a community in which individuals and organizations work together to solve problems and create change (Rappaport, 1987; Sarason, 1984; Schulz, Israel, Zimmerman, & Checkoway, 1995, 1993; Zimmerman, forthcoming).

Some people experience personal transformations as a result of community change. Charles Kieffer (1984) describes several such people and finds that first they feel powerless and alienated from the world ("You feel powerless, you feel helpless"); then an immediate threat or violation of their integrity has sufficient force to spark their initial participation ("No! I'm going to stay here and fight . . . !"); then they develop supportive relationships with an outside organizer or community counterparts in a collective structure that contributes to a more critical understanding of social and political relations ("It was so important that someone cared enough to be there encouraging me, pushing me . . . no matter how afraid I was"); then they sharpen their skills and strengthen their sense of themselves in the political process ("All of a sudden I grew up . . . "); and then finally they view themselves as leaders and search for personally meaningful ways of applying their new abilities and helping others in the community ("It's changed my whole life–personal, professional, everything. My values have changed. Everything has changed").

Empowerment is commonly viewed as a process that operates on a single level of practice. Thus some social workers claim that if a person feels empowered, then empowerment has taken place even if the person has no actual influence in the community. However, there is an emerging notion of empowerment as a process with multiple levels. For example, Gutierrez (1990) reviews the social work literature on empowerment and finds that the goal of empowerment is most often expressed as an increase in personal power, that it tends not to distinguish the individual perception and actual increase in personal power, and that it tends not to reconcile personal and political power. She suggests that the goal of empowerment is not individual but multilevel and concludes: "It is not sufficient to focus only on developing a sense of personal power or working toward social change, but efforts to change should encompass individual, interpersonal, and institutional levels of practice" (p. 152).

Empowerment thus can be viewed as a multilevel process that includes individual involvement, organizational development, and community change. Any one of these elements has potential to serve positive functions. At its best, however, empowerment includes all three of these levels.

MULTICULTURAL, NOT MONOCULTURAL

Community change builds on the notion of community as a form of intervention, but what happens when the community is viewed as multicultural?

In a society in which people seem similar in their social or cultural characteristics, or in which a majority group has dominance over minorities, it is possible to understand the existence of "monocultural" institutions that emphasize assimilation, ignore diversity, or permit powerholders from the dominant coalition to promote the status quo (Crowfoot & Chesler, n.d.; Jackson & Holvino, 1988). As society becomes more socially diverse in the number of "other" groups, however, these changes challenge institutions to recognize differences and reformulate their practice (Daley & Wong, 1994).

Multicultural community change is a process that recognizes the differences between groups while also increasing interaction and cooperation among them. It assumes that there are intrapersonal and interpersonal differences among individuals, intracommunity and intercommunity differences among groups, and opportunities for conflict or collaboration among them. Multicultural community change is neither "culturally-sensitive" practice that makes change more responsive of particular groups (Gutierrez & Lewis, 1992) nor "anti-oppressive" organizing that mobilizes people to deal with their enemies (Crowfoot & Chesler, n.d.), but rather a new form that recognizes differences and builds bridges at the community level (Bradshaw, Soifer, & Gutierrez, 1994).

When the community is viewed as multicultural, it raises questions about each element of the change process. Does the organization represent the social diversity of the community? Do the leaders show commitment to the multicultural mission? Do meetings facilitate the verbal and nonverbal communications differences among groups? These are the types of questions whose answers require new forms of intervention in most communities.

Multiculturalism is neither "normal" nor "politically correct" in societies where prejudice and discrimination prevail, or where people from the majority coalition use their power to prevent their displacement by the growing number of others. It is problematic when the concept of community does not keep up with changes in society.

WHAT ABOUT YOU?

These core concepts provide perspectives on community change as a process of joining together, in solidarity. It includes efforts at starting where people are, awakening the need for action, and developing a structure for change. It views the community as a unit of solution, and community change as an awakening process based upon several strategies and skills.

These concepts are based on a belief that creating community change is an empowering process. It assumes that power is a present or potential resource in every person or community. There is always another community that can become empowered. The key is for people to recognize and act upon the power or potential that they already have.

Core concepts integrate thought and action in a new combination that contributes to the change process. This may seem simplistic, but many people are quick to react to a crisis rather than to reflect upon their principles first. "Take care of the crisis first" is a common notion in professional practice, but it would be as mistaken to act without thought as it is to reflect without taking action.

People would benefit from developing their own core concepts for community change. The concepts expressed here are one version, and cannot substitute for your own formulation. If you question these concepts—which I sincerely hope you will—or substitute your own, my purpose will be served. What are *your* core concepts for community change?

REFERENCES

Alinsky, S. (1969). *Reveille for radicals.* New York: Vintage Books.
Alinsky, S. (1971). *Rules for radicals: A practical primer for realistic radicals.* New York: Vintage.
Bandura, A. (1982). Self-efficacy mechanism in human agency. *American Psychologist, 37*: 122- 47.

Berger, P.J., & J. Neuhaus. (1977). *To empower people: The role of mediating structures in public policy.* Washington: American Enterprise Institute for Public Policy Research.

Biddle, W.W., & L.J. Biddle. (1965). *The community development process: The rediscovery of local initiative.* New York: Holt, Rinehart and Winston.

Bradshaw, C., Soifer, S., & Gutierrez, L. (1994). Toward a hybrid model for effective organizing in communities of color. *Journal of Community Practice, 1(1),* 25-42.

Brown, L.D. (1993). Social change through collective reflection with Asian non-governmental development organizations. *Human Relations, 46,* 249-245.

Catalfo, P. (1993). America online. In S. Walker (Ed.), *Changing community.* St. Paul: Graywolf Press.

Chavis, D.M., & Wandersman, A. (1990). Sense of community in the urban environment: A catalyst for participation and community development. *American Journal of Community Psychology, 18:* 55-81.

Checkoway, B. (1991). *Six strategies of community change.* Jerusalem: The Hebrew University.

Checkoway, B. (Ed.) (1981). *Citizens and health care: Participation and planning for social change.* New York: Pergamon Press.

Checkoway, B., Freeman, H, & Hovaguimian, T. (Eds.) (1988). Community-based initiatives to reduce social isolation and to improve health of the elderly. *Danish Medical Bulletin, 6:* Special Supplement.

Cottrell, L.S. (1993). The competent community. In R. Warren & L. Lyons (Eds.), *New perspectives on the American community.* Homewood: Dorsey Press.

Crowfoot, J., & Chesler, M. (n.d.). *The concept of the enemy: Reflections on the strategic use of language.* Ann Arbor: School of Education.

Daley, J.M., & Wong, P. (1994). Community development with emerging ethnic communities. *Journal of Community Practice, 1(1),* 9-24.

Eng, E. (1988). Extending the unit of practice from the individual to the community. *Danish Medical Bulletin, 6,* 45-52.

Eng, E., & Blanchard, L. (1991). Action-oriented community diagnosis. *International Quarterly of Community Health Education, 11,* 93-110.

Fanon, F. (1968). *The wretched of the earth.* New York: Grove Press.

Freire, P. (1970). *Pedagogy of the oppressed.* New York: Seabury Press.

Garber, J., & Seligman, M. (Eds.), (1980). *Human helplessness: Theory and applications.* New York: Academic Press.

Gatt-Fly, (1983). *AH-HAH! A new approach to popular education.* Toronto: Between the Lines.

Gaventa, J. (1988). Participatory research in America. *Convergence, 21,* 19-27.

Gutierrez, L.M. (1990). Working with women of color: An empowerment perspective. *Social Work, 35,* 149-52.

Gutierrez, L.M., & Lewis, E.A. (1994). Community organizing with women of color: A feminist approach. *Journal of Community Practice, 1(2),* 23-44.

Henderson, P., & Thomas, D.N. (1987). *Skills in neighbourhood work.* London: George Allen and Unwin.

Heskin, A.D., & Heffner, R.A. (1987). Learning about bilingual, multicultural organizing. *The Journal of Applied Behavioral Science, 23*: 525-41.

Hope, A., & Timmel, S. (1984). *Training for transformation: A handbook for community workers.* Gweru, Zimbabwe: Mambo Press.

Horton, M. (1990). *The long haul: An autobiography.* New York: Doubleday.

Horwitt, S.D. (1989). *Let them call me rebel: Saul Alinsky, his life and legacy.* New York: Random House.

Hyde, C. (1994). Commitment to social change: Voices from the feminist movement. *Journal of Community Practice, 1* (2), 45-64.

Iscoe, I. (1974). Community psychology and the competent community. *American Psychologist, 29*, 607-13.

Jackson, B., & Holvina, E. (1988). *Multicultural organization development.* Ann Arbor: Program on Conflict Management Alternatives.

Kahn, S. (1991). *Organizing: A guide for grassroots leaders.* Silver Spring: National Association of Social Workers.

Kasperson, R.E., &. Brietbart, M. (1974). *Participation, decentralization, and advocacy planning.* Washington: Association of American Geographers.

Kendall, J. (1991). *Organizing for social change: A manual for activism in the 1990s.* Washington: Seven Locks Press.

Kieffer, C. (1984). Citizen empowerment: A developmental perspective. *Prevention in Human Services, 3*, 9-36.

Lackey, A.S. (1987). Healthy communities: The goal of community development. *Journal of the Community Development Society, 18*, 1-17.

Marti-Costa, S., & Serrano-Garcia, I. (1987). Needs assessment and community development. In F.M. Cox, J.L. Erlich, J. Rothman, & J.E. Tropman, (Eds.), *Strategies of community organization* (pp. 362-72). Itasca: F.E. Peacock.

McCarthy, J., & Zald, M. (1973). *The trend of social movements in America: professionalization and resource mobilization.* Morristown: General Learning Corporation.

McKnight, J.L., & J. Kretzman. (n.d.). *Mapping community capacity.* Evanston: Center for Urban Affairs and Policy Research.

McMillan, D.W., & Chavis, D.M. (1986). Sense of community: A definition and theory. *Journal of Community Psychology, 14*, 6-23.

Minkler, M. (1990). Improving health through community organization. In K. Glanz, F.M. Lewis, & B.K. Rimen (Eds.). *Health behavior and health education* (pp. 257-87). San Francisco: Jossey-Bass.

Pitkin, H.F. (1969). *Representation.* New York: Atherton Press.

Rappaport, J. (1981). In praise of paradox: A social policy of empowerment over prevention. *American Journal of Community Psychology, 9*, 1-25.

Rappaport, J. (1987). Terms of empowerment/exemplars of prevention: Toward a theory for community psychology. *American Journal of Community Psychology, 15*, 121-44.

Reitzes, D.C., & Reitzes, D.C. (1980). Saul D. Alinsky's contribution to community development. *Journal of the Community Development Society, 11*, 39-5.

Rivera, F. G., & Erlich, J.L. (Eds.), (1992). *Community organizing in a diverse society.* Boston: Allyn and Bacon.

Rothman, J., with J.E. Tropman. (1987). Models of community organization and macro practice perspectives: Their mixing and phasing. In F.M. Cox, J.L. Erlich, J. Rothman & J.E. Tropman (Eds.), *Strategies of community organization* (pp. 3-25). Itasca: F.E. Peacock.

Rubin, H.J., & Rubin, I.S. (1992). *Community organizing and development.* New York: Macmillan.

Ryun, W. (1976). *Blaming the victim.* New York: Vintage Books.

Sarason, S.B. (1984). *The psychological sense of community: Prospects for a community psychology.* San Francisco: Jossey-Bass.

Schon, D. (1983). *The reflective practitioner: How professionals think in action.* New York: Basic Books.

Schulz, A., Israel, B.A., Zimmerman, M.A., & Checkoway, B.N. (1995). Empowerment as a multi-level construct: Perceived control at the individual, organizational and community levels. *Health Education Research, 10,* 309-27.

Speeter, G. (1978). *Power: A repossession manual-organizing strategies for citizens.* Amherst: Citizen Involvement Training Project.

Staples, L. (1984). *Roots to power: A manual for grassroots organizing.* New York: Praeger.

Steuart, G.W. (1993). Social and cultural perspectives: Community intervention and mental health. *Health Education Quarterly, Supplement 1:* S99-12.

Suttles, G.D. (1972). *The social construction of communities.* Chicago: University of Chicago Press.

Tait, J.L. & Bokenheimer, H. (n.d.). *Identifying the community power actors: A guide for change agents.* Ames: Cooperative Extension Service.

Tweeten, L., & Brinkman, G.L. (1976). *Micropolitan development.* Ames: Iowa State University Press.

Unger, D.G., & Wandersman, A. (1985). The importance of neighborhoods: The social, cognitive, and affective components of neighboring. *American Journal of Community Psychology, 13,* 139-70.

Warren, R.L. (1972). *The community in America.* Chicago: Rand McNally.

Webber, M. (1963). Order in diversity: Community without propinquity. In L. Wingo (Ed.), *Cities and space: The future use of urban level.* Baltimore: Johns Hopkins Press.

Werner, D. (1993). *Where there is no doctor.* Palo Alto: The Hesperian Foundation.

Werner, D., & Bower, B. (1983). *Helping health workers learn.* Palo Alto: The Hesperian Foundation.

Zimmerman, M.A. (forthcoming). Empowerment theory: Psychological, organizational and community levels of analysis. In J. Rappaport and E. Seidman (Eds.), *Handbook of community psychology.* New York: Plenum Press.

Zimmerman, M.A. et al. (1992). Further explorations in empowerment theory: An empirical analysis of psychological empowerment. *American Journal of Community Psychology, 20:* 707-727.

Public Life in Gulfton:
Multiple Publics
and Models of Community Organization

Lisa Taaffe, LMSW
Robert Fisher, PhD

SUMMARY. Based on a case study of six community organizations in the Gulfton neighborhood in Houston, Texas, this paper proposes that community organization models need to consider that highly diverse and often contentious community efforts within a single community represent well the context of life in contemporary heterogeneous urban neighborhoods. Despite reservations, we find this diversity of organizational efforts and even the tensions among them generally positive, as they often reflect the most vibrant forms of public life in our otherwise privatizing world. Rethinking the diversity of community organizations as multiple publics in a privatizing context provides new openings for the importance and value of community organization within schools of social work and the larger society. *[Article copies available for a fee from The Haworth Document Delivery Service: 1-800-342-9678. E-mail address: getinfo@haworth.com]*

KEYWORDS. Community organizing, Houston, models of community organizing

---

Lisa Taaffe is Project Manager for Communities in Schools, Houston.

Robert Fisher is Professor and Chair, Political Social Work at the Graduate School of Social Work, University of Houston.

Address correspondence to: Robert Fisher, Graduate School of Social Work, University of Houston, Houston, TX 77204-4492.

[Haworth co-indexing entry note]: "Public Life in Gulfton: Multiple Publics and Models of Community Organization." Taaffe, Lisa, and Robert Fisher. Co-published simultaneously in *Journal of Community Practice* (The Haworth Press, Inc.) Vol. 4, No. 1, 1997, pp. 31-56; and: *Community Practice: Models in Action* (ed: Marie Weil) The Haworth Press, Inc., 1997, pp. 31-56. Single or multiple copies of this article are available for a fee from The Haworth Document Delivery Service [1-800-342-9678, 9:00 a.m. - 5:00 p.m. (EST). E-mail address: getinfo@haworth.com].

31

We increasingly live in a private as opposed to a public world. Public life, Ryan (1992) offers, encourages "open, inclusive, and effective deliberation about matters of common and critical concern" (p. 259). Habermas (1989) further suggests that the public represents what is open to all, as opposed to exclusive or closed affairs, or what is tied to the state, such as a public building, which is not necessarily open to all but which houses the government and is fundamentally about "promoting the public or common welfare of its rightful members" (p. 2). Public life is about the creation and maintenance of society, and existence in a social world larger than one's self or one's family. Public life is life at work, at school, in communities, as citizens of a city, nation, and world. It includes both the public sector and civil society, the world outside of both the public and private sectors. Public life is also the world of contact with acquaintances and strangers–city streets, parks, beaches, buses, libraries–which includes a broad diversity of people.

While some of the key features of the contemporary context–a post-industrial global economy dominated by a politics of neoconservatism–produce a general decline in shared public life and, consequently, a more private world, a highly diverse and often fragmented public life has been developing at the grassroots. The disparate aims of different community groups in a single neighborhood reflect a movement towards organizing based on communities of interest–racial/ethnic/political–as well as communities of place. This trend can be clearly seen in the Gulfton neighborhood of Houston, Texas, where community organizing has flourished in a diverse and fractious community.

Based on a case study of six community organizations in Gulfton, we propose that the proliferation of highly diverse and often contentious community efforts within a single community represents well the nature of contemporary organizing and the context of life in heterogeneous urban neighborhoods. Moreover, despite reservations, we find this diversity and tension generally positive, even as they are difficult and fraught with problems. Diverse, polyvocal, contemporary community organizations serve a critical secondary role of maintaining and invigorating public life. The proliferation of community work not only expands public life, it challenges a common assumption among organizers and theorists about the importance of community unity in advancing neighborhood interests. Mansbridge (1980), for example, presumes a shared, predominant interest of organizations *within* communities; tensions between organizations, what she calls "adversary democracy," are reserved for powers outside the neighborhood. This has always been a central precept of most organizing, within and without social work. Jane Addams sought to unite the neighborhood around Hull House. Saul Alinsky sought to do the same in Back of the Yards. Most community organizing in the 1990s promotes "consensus organizing" strategies to build neighborhood solidarity (Fisher, 1994). Even social work models of community organization practice (Fisher, 1994; Rothman, 1986; Weil & Gamble, 1995) inherently compartmentalize contemporary efforts, rarely addressing how a multiplicity of efforts impacts a single community.

The Gulfton case study[1] which follows suggests that contemporary efforts be viewed in a more postmodern way: not only as subjective entities tied to diverse constituencies, leadership, ideologies and agendas but also as manifestations of the dynamic multiple publics of contemporary public life. In the short-term, these multiple publics seem to undermine the development of a united progressive community agenda—fragmenting social change into countless grassroots efforts. In the long run, by expanding public life and legitimating social claims and needs, they may contribute to the larger social change project of rebuilding public and community life around the ideals of democratic process, cultural diversity, and social struggle.

The case study also suggests that those engaged in studying and organizing communities need to consider how communities and community organizations are affected by such constructs as economic globalization, privatization, postmodernism, and multiculturalism. In a nutshell, we argue that in a postindustrial-oriented global economy dominated by neoconservative politics and fragmented efforts to resist the new political economy, life becomes more private in a three-fold manner. People are (1) increasingly concerned with personal rather than social development (Bellah, Madsen, Sullivan, Swindler, & Tipton, 1985; Lasch, 1991), (2) increasingly located in private rather than public physical spaces (Sorkin, 1992), and (3) increasingly dominated by private rather than public institutions (Barnekov, Boyle, & Rich, 1989). As the world becomes more private, knowledge of economic globalization, privatization, post-modernism, and multiculturalism leads to a different lens for viewing not only contemporary community efforts but also models of community practice. The lens, of course, is not entirely new. For example, the concept of "multiple publics," basic to postmodern theories of resistance, is not new to community organization. The history of community organizing is full of diverse efforts and forms of community organization in single neighborhoods, although the literature about and models of community organization tend to focus heavily on individual organizations rather than multiple efforts in communities. This case study of Gulfton proposes that the diverse efforts of contemporary community life occur in a new context, one altered by these new constructs, which heightens the significance of multiple efforts, their relation to each other, and their contribution to the larger agenda of progressive social change.

GULFTON'S DEVELOPMENT

The Gulfton area of Houston is a 3.2 square mile community, accessible to downtown Houston, with a 1990 demographic break-down of 54% Latino, 21% Anglo, 17% African American, and 9% Asian American (Census Report, 1990). In the 1950s the only development in the Gulfton area was the Shenandoah subdivision, a quiet suburban neighborhood. The glory years of the oil industry in Houston, which began in the late 1950s, ushered in a period of overwhelming growth in Houston. Between the mid-1960s and early 1970s, the Texas economy grew about one and a half times as fast as the national economy (Feagin, 1988; Rodriguez, 1993). As the economy grew, so did the labor force, which necessitated the construction of apartment and industrial complexes. Gulfton, with its easy accessibility to freeways and its proximity to downtown Houston, was a natural target for developers. By the early 1980s it had become largely an apartment enclave for young professionals.

Construction of apartment complexes in Gulfton between 1965 and 1980 occurred partially to accommodate the volume of people moving to Houston and partially for developers to benefit from federal tax incentives for real estate investment (Feagin, 1988).

During the oil boom, the Gulfton apartments were filled with young professionals attracted to Houston's thriving economy. At one point during the 1970s, there were close to 1,000 people per week moving to Houston, and total employment grew by 145% (Fisher, 1989; Rodriguez, 1993). When Houston's economy collapsed in 1982, many of these people left to find jobs elsewhere. The apartment complexes in Gulfton, which had relied precisely on the workers most likely to depart, found it difficult to keep their buildings fully occupied. Rents were reduced. Mile after mile of apartment complexes were put up for auction. Those which changed hands frequently slipped into decay (Cobb, 1988; Hooper, 1982; Rodriguez, 1993; Thomas & Murray, 1991).

Between 1982 and 1983, the first of three large waves of Central American immigrants arrived in Houston. Concurrently, Southeast Asian immigration was increasing and Houston's economy was experiencing a downturn (Rodriguez, 1993). The apartment complexes in Gulfton began marketing their apartments to the newly arriving Latino immigrants. Rents were reduced up to 50%, bilingual staff was hired and English classes were offered in apartment complexes that previously had had no trouble finding "Yuppie" tenants. In addition, many managers and owners, desperate to rent the apartments, did not screen applicants. The result of this restructuring strategy by apartment managers and owners was that the primarily Anglo apartment complexes rapidly changed into a popular residential location for both recent immigrants from all over the world and low-income Houstonians seeking to take advantage of the reduced rents.

Developed originally as a middle-class community, Gulfton did not have adequate infrastructure to support a changing population base. Houston is the classic "free enterprise" city, where business needs and styles dominate, government is kept small, and public social services are minimal. It is a "fee-for-service" city in which those with money can purchase services on the private market and those without resources tend to do without services (Feagin, 1988). Gulfton, for example, had virtually no public transportation, no pocket parks or recreational centers, minimal social services, and few sidewalks. Marston and Towers (1993) assert that reasonable community planning by coalitions of business, real estate, and government must include quality of life factors in any evaluation of areas for their income potential. Gulfton, contrarily, developed in the 1970s and declined in the 1980s as a purely short-term, relatively spontaneous speculative process which focused on producing apartment complexes, nightclubs and warehouses. The lack of zoning laws in free-enterprise Houston permitted developers to build new structures next to the older apartment complexes and single family homes in the Shenandoah subdivision. This haphazard development led to dramatic deterioration in property values once the oil boom busted. By 1988, the area was dubbed the "Gulfton ghetto" (Cobb, 1988; Davis, 1992; GAPS, 1992; Marston and Towers, 1993).

THE COMMUNITY ORGANIZES

The rising crime and the decreasing standard of living in Gulfton led to the organization of new community groups, each representing different, but sometimes overlapping, populations. Until the mid-1980s, the only community organizing in Gulfton was done by the *Shenandoah Civic Association*, which, like other civic associations in Houston, mainly sought to protect property values and maintain the status quo (Fisher, 1994). Beginning in 1985, however, people in Gulfton began organizing around specific needs. In 1985, a group of Salvadoran immigrants formed *CARECEN* (Central American Refugee Center) to advocate for peace in El Salvador and to assist Central Americans with their legal needs. The *Gulfton Area Religious Council* coalesced in late 1988 when churches both inside and outside of Gulfton began to work collaboratively to provide desperately needed social services to people in the area (Francisco Lopez, personal communication, October 12, 1994; Reverend John Collier, personal communication, October 13, 1994).

At approximately the same time, area businesses, apartment owners, and citizens concerned about increasing crime rates formed the *Gulfton Area Action Council* (GAAC) to protect property values and reduce crime in Gulfton. Recognition of the need for health and human services in Gulfton led to the formation of the *Southwest Houston Task Force*, which came together to assess community needs, identify community leadership, and advocate for a community health clinic. In 1992, the *Gulfton Area Neighborhood Organization* (GANO) evolved from the Southwest Houston Task Force to try to realize that group's commitment to community empowerment, to represent the needs of the apartment dwellers and to tackle issues of racism and inequality (GAAC newsletter, 1989; Southwest Houston Task Force mission statement; GANO memo, 1992). All six groups are discussed below (see also Table 1). Alone, they represent diverse models of community organization. As a whole, they represent the polyvocal publics of contemporary life–disparate, dynamic, engaged, overwhelmed by problems, and with uncertain prospects.

Shenandoah Civic Association

The Shenandoah Civic Association was established in 1956 in order to protect the property values of the homes in the Shenandoah subdivision of Houston. Unlike many other cities, Houston does not have zoning. Consequently, homeowners in Houston have had to rely upon deed restrictions, which mainly regulate house construction and prohibit homes from also being used as businesses (Feagin, 1988; Fisher, 1994). Most civic clubs in Houston, numbering more than 800 in 1990, were formed primarily to enforce these deed restrictions, enhance the neighborhood property values through neighborhood beautification projects, and lobby for city services on behalf of the subdivision. Without city or state income taxes in Houston, and with a highly conservative political ideology among business and elected leaders, the city has traditionally provided few social services. Residential suburbs have often had to pay for items like street lights and street repairs. Therefore, while the primary function of the Shenandoah Civic Association has always been the enforcement of neighborhood deed restrictions, group members have also acted as key agents in efforts to obtain scarce city services for the neighborhood.

The rapid changes in the design and demographics of Gulfton in the late 1970s and 1980s profoundly affected the Shenandoah neighborhood. Unregulated development resulted in warehouses, bars, and nightclubs springing up adjacent to the subdivision. Many apartment complex owners who had suffered losses during the economic downturn let their buildings fall into disrepair. This threat-

TABLE 1. Gulfton Community Organizations

ORGANIZATION'S NAME	PRIMARY GOALS	PRIMARY ORGANIZING APPROACH
Central American Refugee Center (CARECEN)	provides legal and some social services, as well as advocacy and publicity for issues of concern to Central American immigrants. Merged with GANO in 1995.[1]	immigrant rights organization; combines advocacy with service delivery.[2]
Gulfton Area Action Council (GAAC)	to restore and revitalize Gulfton, to improve the quality of life and property values in Gulfton and to make the neighborhood safe.[3]	neighborhood maintenance model: maintain neighborhood by fighting threats to property values.[4]
Gulfton Area Neighborhood Organization (GANO)	community empowerment; developing a community-based, comprehensive planning process to solve community problems; protecting civil rights in Gulfton and increasing appreciation of cultural diversity.[5]	multi-racial community organization: community based organization that also: addresses issues not necessarily confined to local community; has formulated an analytical framework based in part on race and race relations; and identifies and trains indigenous leaders.[6]
Gulfton Area Religious Council (GARC)	collaborative, church-based effort to empower the community by helping people meet their medical, social, and educational needs.[7]	locality development model: pursues social justice and economic well-being through consensus building, social integration, & leadership development.[8]
Shenandoah Civic Association	enforcement of deed restrictions, neighborhood beautification, and advocacy in order to protect and enhance the Shenandoah subdivision.[9]	neighborhood maintenance model: (see above)
Southwest Houston Task Force	community needs assessment, leadership identification, advocacy for health clinic.[10]	social planning model: gathers facts to solve problems, implements programs, facilitates process.[11]

1. Francisco Lopez, personal communication, October 12, 1994.
2. Delgado, G. (1994). *Beyond the politics of place: New directions for community organizing the 1990s.* Oakland, CA: Applied Research Center.
3. GAAC newsletter, November 1989.
4. Fisher, R. (1994). Let the people decide: Neighborhood organizing in Houston. New York: Twayne Publishers.
5. GANO Mission Statement (Available from: the Gulfton Area Neighborhood Association, 6006 Bellaire Blvd., Suite 100, Houston, TX 77081).
6. Delgado, G. (1994). *Beyond the politics of place: New directions for community organizing in the 1990s.* Oakland, CA: Applied Research Center.
7. Reverend John Collier, personal communication, October 13, 1994.
8. Rothman, J. (1968). Three models of community organization practice. In F. Cox, J. Erlich, J. Rothman, & J. Tropman (Eds.) *Strategies of community organization: A book of readings* (pp. 3-26). Itasca,IL: Peacock.
9. Shenandoah Shingle (1989, October 9). Shenandoah Civic Association Leader, personal communication, October 26, 1994).
10. Southwest Houston Task Force Mission Statement (Available from: GANO, 6006 Bellaire Blvd., Suite 100, Houston, TX 77081).
11. Rothman, J. (1968). Three models of community organization practice. In F. Cox, J. Erlich, J. Rothman, & J. Tropman (Eds.) *Strategies of community organization: A book of readings* (pp. 3-26). Itasca, IL: Peacock.

ened property values of the single family homes in the Shenandoah area and galvanized the Shenandoah Civic Association (Mike McMahon, personal communication, October 7, 1994; members of Shenandoah Civic Association, personal communication, 1994).

In order to counter the negative effects Gulfton development had on Shenandoah, the civic association established a security patrol, supported efforts to locate a police station in the neighborhood, lobbied the city council to revoke liquor licenses at businesses located around Shenandoah, and engaged in neighborhood beautification projects (Shenandoah Shingle, 1989; Shenandoah Civic Association officer, personal communication, October 26, 1994). While the Shenandoah Civic Association has not been active in addressing problems in the area surrounding their subdivision, they did assist in the advocacy effort that brought Gulfton a neighborhood-based police sub-station. (Called "police storefronts" in Houston, these sub-stations are staffed with fewer officers, are located in apartment complexes or shopping centers, and are supported through community fundraising.) In addition, a number of Shenandoah residents, including the civic association president, supported the formation of a city-funded, day labor hiring hall, a central location where documented and undocumented workers could be hired for day work (Corder, 1993; Shenandoah Shingle, 1991).

Most recently, the civic association has been involved in a controversial city plan to close off streets in Shenandoah. In April of 1992, Houston Mayor Lanier targeted Gulfton as part of a neighborhood revitalization project, one component of which was building barriers around the Shenandoah subdivision, to reduce traffic and subsequently reduce crime. The estimated cost of the project is between $200,000 and $400,000 (Press Release, 1994). The Shenandoah Civic Association is actively pursuing the street closings, feeling that they deserve the protection afforded those living in gated apartment complexes. The other community groups, excluding some GAAC members, oppose the closings, calling them racist, an ineffective way to control crime, a wasteful use of city funds, and bad for local business.

The Shenandoah Civic Association does a good job enforcing deed restrictions and beautifying the neighborhood. Their "neighborhood maintenance" model of community organization (Fisher, 1994), however, is inherently parochial and exclusive. Shenandoah residents try to ignore the Gulfton area surrounding their subdivision, despite the fact that the surrounding area is so critical to property values in Shenandoah. Moreover, despite the fact that the subdivision has become increasingly integrated, civic association members have opposed requests by Latino residents for translators at civic association meetings. Association members' ideas on how to protect their section of the community and enhance their property values turn away from the larger purpose of addressing the needs of the greater community.

Gulfton Area Action Council (GAAC)

The Gulfton Area Action Council (GAAC) is a group of business people who came together in order to reduce the crime and drug problems in Gulfton and to protect property values. It grew out of a town hall meeting called by conservative city council member John Goodner on March 30, 1989, in which people considered what to do about the increasing crime in the area (Mike McMahon, personal communication, October 7, 1994).

In November, 1989, GAAC's first newsletter identified the group's short-term goals. Open a police storefront in Gulfton. Involve the business community. Rid the area of drifters and drug dealers. Initiate landscaping and clean-up in the area. It also devised long-term goals. Restore the neighborhood. Improve the quality of life. Promote higher property values and a safer neighborhood (GAAC newsletter, 1989). To reduce crime and drugs in the neighborhood and to preserve property values, GAAC's strategy primarily focuses on law enforcement. To date, GAAC's greatest success has been getting a police storefront opened in June of 1990. Money was allocated through the city council for a storefront in every council district, but the funds provided by the city were insufficient to staff and furnish the police storefront. GAAC raised funds from area businesses and Shenandoah donated chairs, desks, telephones and coffee. GAAC's other accomplishment has been the transformation of its monthly meetings into an information-sharing forum. GAAC's meetings have provided an opportunity for different groups in the area to share what they have been doing and what they believe needs to be done (Mike McMahon, personal communication, October 7, 1994; SCA member, personal communication, October 21, 1994; SCA officer, personal communication, October 26, 1994; Shenandoah Shingle, 1990).

These types of activities are representative of business-initiated community organization efforts (Fisher, 1994; Rothman, 1986; Weil & Gamble, 1995). Such business-led efforts tend to fear progressive social change and leaders. Six months after its formation, GAAC was successful in getting a police storefront in Gulfton. However, it lost the momentum of this early success by not following it up with other projects. GAAC vetoed participating in advocacy efforts for a community health clinic as well as a survey of the Gulfton area conducted by professors and students at the University of Houston and Rice University. Participation in either or both of these projects would have increased GAAC's credibility within the community in addition to giving GAAC a project in the interim between the storefront and the next endeavor.

Like most neighborhood maintenance efforts, organizations like GAAC tend to be highly exclusive. When asked to broaden its mission and board to be more representative of the diverse groups in the community, GAAC's board refused (GAAC Board minutes, 1992). Like the Shenandoah Civic Association, GAAC has been short-sighted in pursuing primarily law enforcement strategies to reduce crime. Many in the Latino community do not trust any officials, especially the police, and often with good reason. If GAAC is to explore alternative strategies to reduce crime and protect property values, it will need feedback and participation from a broader representation of the community.

Some GAAC board members envision GAAC as a community information-sharing resource. This is an exciting concept, as the community needs to improve intergroup communication, and an impartial entity mediating between opposing organizations would be helpful. However, the conservative politics of GAAC has limited its role in serving *all* groups in the community. GAAC meetings have not always been impartial and some GAAC members have strongly expressed resistance to working with the Gulfton Area Neighborhood Organization (GANO) and some of the Gulfton Area Religious Council (GARC) churches. In addition, during monthly meetings some GAAC members have made openly racist comments or negative allusions about the Latino population in Gulfton (Taggart, January 26, 1994; Francisco Lopez, personal communication, October 12, 1994; Reverend Alessandro Montes, personal communication, October 7, 1994; Reverend Eduardo Cabrera, personal communication, October 7, 1994; Xiomara Cabrera, personal communication, October 13, 1994).

Gulfton Area Religious Council (GARC)

The Gulfton Area Religious Council (GARC) was formed in 1988 by a group of people representing various religious institutions. GARC began when members of the United Methodist Church in the affluent West University area of Houston decided to form a work project to assist a less affluent community. The demographic changes occurring in Gulfton caught their eye and a newspaper article written by the principal of a Gulfton elementary school convinced the church members to assist Gulfton residents. Reverend John Collier and Dr. Peggy Rice of United Methodist arranged a meeting with Reverend Montes of Saint Matthew's Episcopal Church and Sister Juana of Holy Ghost Catholic Church, two of the more active churches in the community. The four agreed to recruit other churches that would work cooperatively on projects in the community (Reverend John Collier, personal communication, October 13, 1994; Reverend Alessandro Montes, personal communication, October 7, 1994; Sister Juana, personal communication, October 12, 1994).

Membership in GARC is open to any Christian church. GARC's mission is to empower the community by helping people meet their medical, social, and educational needs. It proposes to do this by collectively participating in advocacy and by involving its congregations in projects that benefit the community. Since its inception, GARC has engaged in numerous projects in the Gulfton area. It advocated for the establishment of a Head Start program and played a valuable role in the neighborhood effort to bring a city health clinic to Gulfton. In addition, it has been involved in numerous charity efforts, such as finding a volunteer dental hygienist to check teeth at the local elementary school and getting congregations to build bookcases for school libraries (Reverend John Collier, personal communication, October 13, 1994).

GARC's charity efforts have helped alleviate the stresses of poverty, and its advocacy work for a community health clinic proved valuable. Moreover, in the process of identifying and assisting people to meet their basic needs, GARC aims to develop local leadership and to promote community empowerment. This strategy seems to have worked, as GARC membership has grown and GARC activities proliferated.

Of course, by narrowing membership to Christian churches, GARC has also not been inclusive. There are large non-Christian Asian and African populations in Gulfton. Reflecting the limits of the "social work" model of neighborhood organization (Fisher, 1994), GARC has been so involved in ameliorating the conditions of poverty that it has failed to attack its systemic causes. Nevertheless, recent GARC activities indicate that the organization is evolving from a primarily charity organization to a social justice organization. For example, GARC has been active in promoting citizenship and has assisted in organizing protests and marches for immigrant rights. In addition, GARC has begun to involve the community in its efforts. By redirecting its efforts towards community empowerment and community advocacy, GARC is beginning to resemble a "social action" organization (Rothman, 1986).

The Central American Refugee Center (CARECEN)

The Central American Refugee Center (CARECEN) was formed in 1985 by a group of Salvadorans who had recently arrived in Houston. Unlike more conservative immigrant groups, many Salvadorans came to Houston with vast organizing experience and a left politics. Between 1988 and 1992, CARECEN, which provides legal services to immigrants, initially worked with the Central American Refugee Committee to organize people in the community around issues of immigration rights and peace in El Salvador. In Houston, the need for community awareness of the plight of Central American refugees was extremely important during this time, as Central Americans were fleeing their countries and arriving in Texas in large numbers. The need to inform and correct misinformation about Central Americans has been a crucial and on-going part of

CARECEN's work. After peace in El Salvador was reached in 1992, CARECEN expanded its vision and worked to empower the Salvadoran community in Houston. CARECEN continued to provide legal services while also campaigning for the permanent residency of Salvadorans and engaging in ongoing advocacy and publicity regarding issues of concern to Central American immigrants.

CARECEN's most apparent strength has been its ability to adapt its mission to meet the changing needs of the community. In addition, CARECEN is an example of how a social service agency can also be a social justice organization. In Lord and Kennedy's model (1992), a social service/social justice agency meets both the immediate needs of people and involves itself in the political needs of the community. Hyde (1992) refers to groups like CARECEN as social movement agencies, blending political activism with service delivery. CARECEN's strength has been its clarity of purpose and adaptability. In January, 1995, because of overlapping board members and a shared commitment to social justice, CARECEN merged with GANO. This merger with the progressive GANO, which opposed the controversial neighborhood street closings, makes less likely work with the more conservative organizations, the Shenandoah Civic Association and GAAC.

The Southwest Houston Task Force

The Southwest Houston Task Force was a coalition of representatives from the health and human services, city government, religious institutions, businesses, schools and Gulfton residents. Its mission was to identify and address needs at the community level, improve coordination of community resources, educate the community about the changing needs and services in Southwest Houston, and assist in the implementation of health and human services in Southwest Houston (Southwest Houston Task Force mission statement).

The task force evolved from two initial meetings of community groups and representatives of the city in regard to bringing a city health clinic to Gulfton. The meetings brought quick results (Sorell, 1989). The Sisters of Charity Southwest Health Clinic, operated jointly with the City of Houston, opened in June of 1991. It was the area's first large scale health care clinic, providing pre-natal and child health care, especially immunizations and TB screening. Once this was accomplished, the Southwest Houston Task Force lost its focal issue. The group did a community needs assessment, identified some local leaders in early 1992, and then disbanded.

Task focused, like most "social planning" types of community organization, the Southwest Houston Task Force was successful in its primary goal of getting a health care clinic located in Gulfton. In the process, it identified community leaders, conducted a needs assessment, and honed the advocacy skills of the people who got involved. Most of the participants in the Southwest Task Force were from outside the community and most were professionals, academics, and/or representatives of the city. To its credit, the group recognized this and committed itself to locating existing leaders and developing indigenous leadership in the community. Through this process, Mike McMahon of GAAC and Francisco Lopez of CARE-CEN met. When the Southwest Houston Task Force dispersed, Francisco and Mike joined forces to form the Gulfton Area Neighborhood Organization.

Gulfton Area Neighborhood Organization (GANO)

The Gulfton Area Neighborhood Organization (GANO) was formed in August of 1992. GANO's founders hoped to continue the preliminary efforts at community empowerment initiated by the Southwest Houston Task Force and to create a group that was more inclusive and representative of the diverse needs and visions of the whole community than GAAC. The conditions in many of the apartment complexes at the time were unbearable, yet no one was advocating for the needs of the apartment residents. Mike McMahon proposed to GAAC that the group expand its mission to represent the entire community and address a broad array of problems, including, but not limited to, education and health care. The board voted against this proposal. McMahon resigned and helped form GANO to meet these larger goals (GAAC Board minutes, 1992; Mike McMahon, personal communication, October 7, 1992).

GANO has been a very active community organization. Some of its projects include: starting an adult and a youth soccer league, becoming involved in the university-related Gulfton Area Plan Survey (GAPS) project, successfully advocating for increased METRO bus routes in the Gulfton area, establishing of the Day Labor Center, sponsoring consumer credit counseling, initiating a rights aware- ness program for apartment residents and non-union workers, and embarking upon a citizenship campaign. GANO's strategy is to improve the quality of life by empowering the community, by involving residents in decisions that effect their lives, by protecting civil rights, and by coordinating and implementing programs and services. GANO has employed a variety of tactics: they have marched and protested, trained and educated, and advocated and publicized (Francisco Lopez, personal communication, October 12, 1994; Mike McMahon, personal communication, October 7, 1992; GANO minutes, 1992-1994).

Like most comparable community organizing efforts, GANO tries to accomplish too much with too few resources. The problem conditions in the neighborhood seem to demand it. With only two paid staff members (prior to its merger with CARECEN), it orga- nized against the street closings, started a basketball pavilion, advo- cated for the multi-service center, ran citizenship classes, and helped University interns initiate three separate coalitions with pub- lic schools, businesses, and health care agencies.[2] This was in addi- tion to ongoing projects such as worker rights education and the soccer league, and the numerous other responsibilities handled by Mike McMahon and Francisco Lopez, who are not paid for their work at GANO. GANO and CARECEN's merger in January, 1995, has increased the number of projects in which GANO is involved, while at the same time inevitably identifying GANO increasingly as a "Latino" organization. While GANO has been very successful, its future success depends upon its ability to recognize its limits or mobilize additional social change resources.

THE DIVERSITY OF ORGANIZING IN GULFTON

The different approaches and configurations of neighborhood groups in Gulfton suggest that any expectation of a united commu- nity is unrealistic. Their politics, goals, ideology, and constituencies are as varied as the neighborhood. For example, the Gulfton Area Action Council (GAAC) and the Shenandoah Civic Association embody Fisher's (1994) depiction of neighborhood maintenance organizations: conservative, primarily composed of middle class people and engaged in efforts to maintain the neighborhood and property values. The Gulfton Area Religious Council (GARC) has changed over time, reflecting Fisher's (1994) social work approach and Rothman's (1986) three models: locality development, social planning, and social action. GARC primarily pursues social justice and economic well-being through consensus building, social integration, and leadership development. CARECEN, like other immigrant rights organizations (Delgado, 1994), combines advocacy for Central American immigrants with service delivery. CARECEN could also be considered a "functional community" (Weil & Gamble, 1995), as its members share a common desire for social justice for Latinos that extends beyond Gulfton's borders. The Gulfton Area Neighborhood Organization's (GANO) organizing style most closely resembles Delgado's (1994) conceptualization of a "multiracial community organization," which will: (1) address issues not necessarily confined to local communities (i.e., El Salvador or Proposition 187); (2) formulate an analytical framework based on race and race relations; and (3) identify and train indigenous organizers (Delgado, 1994).

When viewed individually some of the groups in Gulfton appear exclusive and resistant to public discourse about community problems. But, the diversity of interests and community groups is exactly what makes Gulfton a politicized neighborhood. The homeowners have a voice. The business owners have a voice. The churches provide a vehicle for community involvement. The apartment dwellers and Latinos have opportunities to become involved in the political activities of their neighborhood. The tensions between the groups adds to the vitality of public life in Gulfton. People get involved to defend their turf, advance their interests, build community, and unite with others to the extent possible. For example, in November of 1995 a grant to the Gulfton community from the Texas State Legislature to create a prevention-based proposal to reduce juvenile crime rates prompted GANO/CARECEN to work together with Shenandoah and GARC. Community unity on this project, even among contentious groups, was aided because these groups were already organized and active. While community

unity is an exception in Gulfton, the problems the neighborhood faces makes the quantity of organized activity that much more important. The social issues and tensions being played out in Gulfton have created a highly politicized and dynamic public life that helps the community, but does not create the unified neighborhood activity envisaged by Mansbridge (1980).

Community organization in Gulfton is highly illustrative of the diverse publics of contemporary life and supportive of the postmodern conceptualization of community organization (Fisher & Kling, 1993). As Kaufmann (1990) puts it, the "proliferation of multiple publics" reflects the "postmodernization of public life" (p. 10). The more centering narratives of social change (e.g., Marxist and class-based organizing) and centering forms of organizational structure (e.g., the industrial city and union organizing) give way to more decentered, polyvocal social change efforts organized around single issues and the politics of culture and identity. The fact that distinctively different organizations work together, as they did recently for the Gulfton Youth Development Grant and as GANO and the Civic Association did in raising money for the police storefront and advocating for the Day Labor Center, becomes less essential than the fact that the varied groups continue to mobilize interest and heighten consciousness in Gulfton. Of course, multiple community organization efforts have always occurred in single neighborhoods. But this case study proposes that the diverse efforts of contemporary community life occur in a new context that alters the significance of multiple efforts, their relation to each other, and their contribution to the larger agenda of progressive social change. Because globalization and privatization increasingly undermine the public world and because postmodernism and multiculturalism inform those interested in social change of the importance of diverse voices and perspectives, the cumulative effect of all the organizations in Gulfton, in advancing both public life and social change reflective of the diversity of the Gulfton community, may be as significant as their individual accomplishments.

This case study does not propose that all efforts are of equal value in the cause of progressive social change or that building unity among progressive organizing efforts is not a major task for the future. Rather, in an era dominated by reactionary agendas that seek to push people and discourse into purely private matters, the vibrancy and range of community organization activity and political debate in Gulfton, in a city known for its quiescent political culture (Feagin, 1988), demands a rethinking of community organization theory and models as well as social change in our contemporary context. At the least it proposes a more inclusive approach, which addresses the complementary nature of diverse organizing efforts in the cause of social change and the larger agenda of expanding "public life" that community efforts, intentionally or not, help to advance.

IMPLICATIONS FOR SOCIAL WORK PRACTICE AND COMMUNITY ORGANIZATION EDUCATION

Little that happens in local communities these days is not affected by the dramatic changes occurring in the global economy. The new global economy is characterized by an increased velocity and competitiveness of transnational capital in a world undergoing profound technological changes. It is also characterized by global pressures for a more private society, as public life, such as social services or social movements, adds social costs and thereby diminishes private profits, agendas, and power. For our purposes, there are two central features of the new global political economy and the postmodern resistances to it, of which activity in Gulfton is an excellent example. First, the postindustrial economy yields communities that are more fluid and diverse than the unified and stable communities associated with an industrial political economy. Compare, for example, the Back of the Yards neighborhood in the 1930s to Gulfton in the 1990s (Fisher, 1994; Horwitt, 1990). Second, the neoconservative program to dismantle and delegitimize the public sector, and the fragmentation of organizational groups around single issues and cultural identity rather than neighborhood or place, leads to the wide proliferation of grassroots responses to address social problems. At the very moment that the global economy and neoconservative policy destabilize communities, they push the solution to social problems onto them. Increasingly, because of the general absence of government leadership and the decline of centering ideologies of social change, community life becomes more and more contested and conflictual despite attempts to unite and moderate community organizations. Under these new conditions, community organization becomes a major form of public life; it becomes a primary forum for the discussion of social problems and strategies to solve them. We presume that this development should begin to be reflected in a heightened interest in community organization among social work educators, students, and programs.

Community organization is important to *all* social work because it inherently links practice to its social and political context. During the past 20 years there has been a decline in the importance and salience of community organization within the profession. The increasing shift towards psychotherapeutic interventions (Specht & Courtney, 1994) decontextualizes individual problems and promotes decontextualized individual-based solutions with little consideration given to the macro contexts of neighborhood, community, organizations, and the larger political economy. These contexts, however, inform and explain the significance and reality of individual problems.

The current low ebb of community organization within schools of social work and within agencies comes at an inopportune time when the context for social work practice is not only becoming much worse (Fabricant & Burghardt, 1992; Fisher & Karger, forthcoming) but changing so rapidly and dramatically as to require fresh conceptualizations of community organization and more contextualized conceptions of social work in general. We would argue that community organization can play a leading role in recontextualizing social work practice by examining closely the changes in our contemporary macro context and revising community organization theory and models accordingly. This project has already begun (Delgado, 1994; Gutierrez & Lewis, 1995; Hyde, 1989; Mondros & Wilson, 1994; Weil & Gamble, 1995).

The importance of public life in an increasingly private world needs to be added to the debate. This paper has argued that in a postindustrial global economy dominated by neoconservative politics and fragmented contemporary resistances, there is a general decline of shared public life and an increasing emphasis on the private individual, private space, and private sector. The decontextualization of social work and the shift away from community organization in social work education are manifestations of this phenomenon. We propose that the very practice of *social* work depends on countering the shift to an increasingly private world, and that schools of social work are well situated to do this. As Hanna and Robinson (1994) argue in their examination of organizing training institutes outside of schools of social work, it is the training of community organizers inside schools of social work where a larger understanding of context, theory, history, and policy occurs. Training institutes are too brief to focus on much more than skills and a single model of organizing. Schools of social work have the time and mission to immerse students in a critical understanding and evaluation of social conditions and solutions. Given the vast changes evident in our contemporary context, community organization in schools of social work needs to be expanded to effectively reinstill the *social* in social work training and provide the necessary broad understanding of contemporary change critical to community organizing training in and outside of the academy.

CONCLUSION

Certainly the current aspects of community fragmentation have made the reality of multiple publics more visible. The consequences of these changes, however, are yet to be fully revealed. Will they result in more social change and social actors–a new dynamic public life that empowers more citizens and raises critical consciousness? Or will contemporary multiple publics fragment resistances and permit the corporate lords of the new global economy to rule virtually unchallenged? In this era of dramatic changes in urban life and political economy–comparable to those that accompanied the industrial revolution of the late 19th century in the United States– prospects for the new multiple publics are uncertain. Gulfton is filled with democratic potential, but limited by virtue of its small scale and scope in the face of massive problems, most of which derive from outside the neighborhood. Because struggle forms more and more around specific community issues and cultural identification, models of community organization must incorporate the postmodern emphasis on diverse and disunited communities with more unifying conceptualizations such as class and place. As Martin Hernandez describes of his organizing work for the Los Angeles

Bus Riders Union, the buses are "factories on wheels. . . . Since deindustrialization, buses are among the last public spaces where blue collar people of all races still mingle" (Davis, 1995, p. 272). Similarly, Brecher and Costello (1994) call for a globalization of the grassroots in which community organizations build transnational organizations around issues such as environmental destruction or the North Atlantic Free Trade Agreement (NAFTA), which not only connect local concerns to each other but also to the struggle over the goals of the global economy.

In terms of future research regarding theories and models of community organization and the potential contribution of community organization research to contemporary social theory, the Gulfton case study contradicts two of the key elements of the postmodern model of contemporary grassroots change, which suggests a decline in the salience of place as the locus of community organizing and an emphasis on "postmaterialist" concerns (Delgado, 1994; Fisher & Kling, 1993). Gulfton efforts are rooted in culture as well as place. Invisible, however, are the "postmaterialist" groupings–around gender, sexual orientation, and environmental issues, for example–that are said to characterize the "turn to culture" and the focus on quality, rather than quantity, of life. In Gulfton, economic issues and needs continue to dominate. Materialist objectives of the affluent and poor take center stage in a neoconservative political economy which throws issues of basic survival back onto citizens and neighborhoods. In Gulfton, we find a tight linkage between issues of culture (ethnicity, religion, etc.) and class/materialist needs (property values, basic services, etc.). Class may have less significance in traditionally more affluent cultural communities (e.g., environmental, feminist, gay, and peace groupings), or in many nations of Western Europe where social democratic regimes addressed basic social needs. But in poor or heterogeneous communities like Gulfton in the United States, or in most communities composed largely of Third World people, whether they now reside in the Southern or Northern hemisphere, class inequality and basic material human needs remain essential to community work. In this way, despite the more contemporary form of diverse multiple publics in a single community, older models of essentially class-based social action interweave in Gulfton with recent postmodern conceptualizations concerned with culture and quality of life. The contemporary context may be new and demanding of revised models of social change, but class remains a critical component of current community organizing.

Lastly, the Gulfton case study directs us to focus on the issue of public life in an increasingly private world (Fisher & Karger, forthcoming). New theories of community organizing might emphasize less whether organizing should occur around issues of place (neighborhood and workplace) or cultural identity (race, gender, sexual orientation, etc.). Instead, greater attention could be paid to whether organizing occurs around collective issues in public spaces that expand the public realm, public discourse, and public participation or whether it focuses on exclusive private needs and concerns which turn individuals, organizations, and communities inward and away from public life. An emphasis on the importance of expanding public life in an increasingly private world, and its local as well as global implications, offers new insights and potential strategies for students and practitioners of community organization.

NOTES

1. For an impressive treatment of the continued importance and validity of the case study method to social science research see: Feagin, Joe R., Orum, Anthony M., and Sjoberg, Gideon [eds] (1991). *A Case for the Case Study.* Chapel Hill/London: The University of North Carolina Press.

2. While the GAPS project is, to date, the only formal collaborative effort between Houston universities and Gulfton community members, Houston universities have been involved in social change in Gulfton through the placement of interns in the community. GANO has invited field placement students from the University of Texas School of Public Health and the University of Houston Graduate School of Social Work to assist them, most recently, in forming coalitions, researching the history of the neighborhood, and advocating for the community. In return, Gulfton residents and community leaders have shared their time and expertise in university-initiated concerns, such as the Future's Conference and the Inter-Ethnic Forum at the University of Houston.

REFERENCES

Barnekov, T., Boyle, R., & Rich, D. (1989). *Privatism and urban policy in Britain and the United States.* New York: Oxford University Press.

Bellah, R., Madsen, R., Sullivan, W., Swidler, A., & Tipton, S. (1985). *Habits of the heart: Individualism and commitment in American life.* New York: Harper & Row Publishers.

Brecher, J. & Costello, T. (1994). *Global village or global pillage: Economic reconstruction from the bottom up.* Boston: South End Press.

Census Report (1990). (Available from: The Gulfton Area Neighborhood Organization, 6006 Bellaire Boulevard, Ste. 100, Houston, TX 77081.)

Cobb, K. (1988, July 17). Drugs, neglect transform 'single scene' to slums. *Houston Chronicle*, p. 1.

Corder, R. (1993, April 17). Center a step in the right direction [Letter to the editor]. *Houston Chronicle*, p. 11.

Davis, M. (1995, September 18). L.A.'s transit apartheid. *The Nation*, p. 272.

Davis, M. (1992). *City of quartz: Excavating the future in Los Angeles.* New York: Vintage Books.

Delgado, G. (1994). *Beyond the politics of place: New directions for community organizing in the 1990's.* Oakland, CA: Applied Research Center.

Fabricant, M.B., & Burghardt, S. (1992). *The welfare state crisis and the transformation of social service work.* Armonk, NY: M.E. Sharpe.

Feagin, J. (1988). *Free enterprise city: Houston in the political-economic perspective.* New Brunswick and London: Rutgers University Press.

Fisher, R. (1989). Urban policy in Houston, Texas. *Urban Studies, 26,* 144-154.

Fisher, R. (1994). *Let the people decide: Neighborhood organizing in Houston.* New York: Twayne Publishers.

Fisher, R. & Karger, H. (1996). *Getting out in public: Social work and community in a private world.* New York: Longmans.

Fisher, R. & Kling, J. (Eds.) (1993). *Mobilizing the community: Local politics in the era of the global city.* Newbury Park: Sage Publishers.

GAAC Board minutes. (1992, July 14). (Available from: The Gulfton Area Neighborhood Organization, 6006 Bellaire Boulevard, Ste. 100, Houston, TX 77081.)

GAAC newsletter. (1989, November). (Available from: The Gulfton Area Neighborhood Organization, 6006 Bellaire Boulevard, Ste. 100, Houston, TX 77081.)

GANO memo. (1992, August 26). (Available from: The Gulfton Area Neighborhood Organization, 6006 Bellaire Boulevard, Ste. 100, Houston, TX 77081.)

GANO minutes. (1992 - 1994). (Available from: The Gulfton Area Neighborhood Organization, 6006 Bellaire Boulevard, Ste. 100, Houston, TX 77081.)

GAPS report. (1992). (Available from: The Gulfton Area Neighborhood Organization, 6006 Bellaire Boulevard, Ste. 100, Houston, TX 77081.)

Gutiérrez, L., & Lewis, E. (1995). A feminist perspective on organizing with women of color. In: F. Rivera & J. Erlich (Eds). *Community organizing in a diverse society.* 2nd edition. Boston: Allyn and Bacon.

Habermas, J. (1989). *The structural transformation of the public sphere.* Boston: Harvard University Press.

Hanna, M., & Robinson, B. (1994). *Strategies for community empowerment.* Lewiston, NY: The Edwin Mellen Press.

Hooper, C. (1982, October 28). Some apartment complexes in Houston are reducing rents. *Houston Post*, p. 1.

Horwitt, S.D. (1990). *Let them call me rebel: Saul Alinsky–His life and legacy.* New York: Alfred A. Knopf.

Hyde, C. (1989). A feminist model for macro-practice: Promises and problems. *Administration in Social Work (13),* 145-181.

Hyde, C. (1992). The ideational system of social movement agencies. In Y. Hasenfeld (Ed), *Human services as complex organizations* (pp. 121-144). Newbury Park: Sage Publications.

Kaufmann, L.A. (1990, Fall). Democracy in a postmodern world. *Social Policy,* 6-11.

Lasch, C. (1991). *The true and only heaven.* New York: W.W. Norton.

Lord, S., & Kennedy, E. (1992). Transforming a charity organization into a social justice community center. *Journal of Progressive Human Services, 3* (1). pp. 21-37.

Mansbridge, J. (1980). *Beyond adversary democracy.* New York: Basic Books.

Marston, S.A., & Towers, G. (1993). Private spaces and the politics of places: Spatioeconomic restructuring and community organizing in Tucson and El Paso. In: R. Fisher & J. Kling (Eds). *Mobilizing the community: Local politics in the era of the global city* (pp. 75-102). Newbury Park: Sage Publishers.

Mondros, J.B., & Wilson, S.M. (1994). *Organizing for power and empowerment.* New York: Columbia University Press.

Press Release. (1994). re: street closings. (Available from: The Gulfton Area Neighborhood Organization, 6006 Bellaire Boulevard, Ste. 100, Houston, TX 77081.)

Ryan, M. (1992). Gender and public access: Women's politics in nineteenth century America. In C. Calhoun (Ed.), *Habermas and the public sphere* (pp. 259-288). Boston: M.I.T. Press.

Rodriguez, N. (1993). Economic restructuring and Latino growth in houston. In J. Moore, & R. Pinderhughes (Eds). *In the barrios: Latinos and the underclass debate* (pp. 101-127). New York, NY: Russell Sage Foundation.

Rothman, J. (1986). Three models of community organization practice. In F. Cox, J. Ehrlich, J. Rothman, and J. Tropman (eds.). *Strategies of community organization: A book of readings* (pp. 3-26). Itasca, IL: F.E. Peacock.

Shenandoah Shingle (1989, October 9). (Available from: The Gulfton Area Neighborhood Organization, 6006 Bellaire Boulevard, Ste. 100, Houston, TX 77081.)

Shenandoah Shingle (1990, April 7). (Available from: The Gulfton Area Neighborhood Organization, 6006 Bellaire Boulevard, Ste. 100, Houston, TX 77081.)

Shenandoah Shingle (1991, September 9). (Available from: The Gulfton Area Neighborhood Organization, 6006 Bellaire Boulevard, Ste. 100, Houston, TX 77081.)

Sorell, Ruth (1989, November 24). Plan to offer public health facilities for southwest area indigent pledged. *Houston Chronicle,* p. 33.

Sorkin, M. [ed] (1992). *Variation on a theme park: The new American city and the end of public space.* NY: Noonday Press.

Southwest Houston Task Force mission statement. (Available from: The Gulfton Area Neighborhood Organization, 6006 Bellaire Boulevard, Ste. 100, Houston, TX 77081.)

Specht, H., & Courtney, M. (1994). *Unfaithful angels: How social work abandoned its mission.* NY: The Free Press.

Taggart, L. (1994, January 26). Letter to GANO. (Available from: The Gulfton Area Neighborhood Organization, 6006 Bellaire Boulevard, Ste. 100, Houston, TX 77081.)

Thomas, R.D., & Murray, Richard W. (1991). *Progrowth politics.* University of California at Berkley: Institute of Governmental Studies Press.

Weil, M.O. & Gamble, D. (1995). *Community practice models.* In: Encyclopedia of Social Work, 19th edition. MD: NASW.

Being a Conscience and a Carpenter: Interpretations of the Community-Based Development Model

Herbert J. Rubin, PhD

SUMMARY. Though successful in providing affordable housing and employment opportunities within communities of deprivation, community-based development organizations–CBDOs–are criticized by both the activist left and social service scholars. The former claim that CBDOs ignore advocacy work; the latter, that CBDOs minimize social service efforts. Using case study material, this article argues the opposite: community-based development organizations succeed by linking together developmental, advocacy, and social service practices. *[Article copies available for a fee from The Haworth Document Delivery Service: 1-800-342-9678. E-mail address: getinfo@haworth.com]*

KEYWORDS. Community development, CDC, CBDO, neighborhood development, social ideologies, organic theories

Community-based development organizations–CBDOs–are neighborhood-based, non-profit organizations that build affordable housing and create employment opportunities within communities of deprivation. Their very successes, however, engender debate among

---

Herbert J. Rubin is Professor of Sociology at Northern Illinois University.

Address correspondence to: Herbert J. Rubin, Department of Sociology, Northern Illinois University, DeKalb, IL 60115.

[Haworth co-indexing entry note]: "Being a Conscience and a Carpenter: Interpretations of the Community-Based Development Model." Rubin, Herbert J. Co-published simultaneously in *Journal of Community Practice* (The Haworth Press, Inc.) Vol. 4, No. 1, 1997, pp. 57-90; and: *Community Practice: Models in Action* (ed: Marie Weil) The Haworth Press, Inc., 1997, pp. 57-90. Single or multiple copies of this article are available for a fee from The Haworth Document Delivery Service [1-800-342-9678, 9:00 a.m. - 5:00 p.m. (EST). E-mail address: getinfo@haworth.com].

academics (Stoecker, 1994; 1995) and activists (Delgado, 1994) alike. These critics argue that physical development work reduces efforts at advocacy and distracts from social service activities, a concern echoed in standard discussions of models of community practice (Rothman, 1968; Rubin & Rubin, 1992).

Scholars and activists claim differences between the values of the development model and those that guide neighborhood advocacy organizations. They contend, for instance, that CBDOs ignore "empowerment" and instead opt for "economic efficiency," and they argue that CBDO directors choose a "bottom-line business pragmatism" rather then working to promote "neighborhood-controlled social change."

Critics reason that to obtain investment capital from financial institutions, CBDOs brush aside an "advocacy agenda" (Lenz, 1988). Rather than empowering community members, CBDOs become "new rulers in the ghetto" (Berndt, 1977) and act as a conservatizing force that demobilizes neighborhood action. For instance, Randy Stoecker describes that after a neighborhood advocacy organization he studied started development work, its "identity began to shift toward convergence with the conservative community" while "transformative populism within [the organization] ebbed" (Stoecker, 1995, p. 121).

As part of a project examining the community development movement, I explored these value conflicts (Rubin, 1993a; 1993b; 1994; 1995a). Over a three year period, I interviewed leaders of 60 community-based development organizations, as well as activists in trade and technical assistance organizations that help community developers. I was not asking how often CBDOs succeeded (research already done by Vidal, 1989). Rather I was questioning about the models followed by exemplary CBDOs that others could imitate. With this research agenda, I selected five dozen organizations known for either their innovative projects or a steadfast determination to rebuild a neighborhood.

I visited community projects, observed conferences of activists in the community development movement, and conducted 250 open-ended interviews with directors of the CBDOs, core employees, and others who support community development. The material was coded into a database containing about 2 million words and hundreds of documents.

My goal was to learn how and why development organizations undertook the projects they chose. I anticipated hearing about financing, leasing, and physically maintaining buildings. But I also heard from these developmental activists detailed narratives and philosophical ruminations justifying the choices they made.

Developmental activists admitted that the problems pointed out by critics are real. They shared stories of community-based development organizations being co-opted by banks or for-profit developers and described organizations so concerned about economic survival that they abandoned efforts at social change. These activists recognized the tensions between development, advocacy, and social services, yet, in their interviews explained how they reconciled the three approaches.

The developmental activists argued that the dialectic of doing projects requires CBDOs to merge social service efforts and advocacy with physical development. They asserted that to ignore the social service needs of individuals they serve would be to doom physical development projects to rapid destruction, and that without advocacy and lobbying efforts, the entire community development movement would die. Further they explained the logic behind their reasoning by presenting an organic theory detailing how to obtain community empowerment.

My initial plans for interviewing were to learn how developmental activists worked as the carpenters within communities of the poor. Their responses convinced me that developmental activists are also consciences within their communities. Their organizations advocate for changes through which both individuals and communities become empowered by gaining a material stake in the broader society.

In this paper, I build upon quoted words of the developmental activists (Rubin & Rubin, 1995) to describe how they reconcile development work with both social service and advocacy efforts. The examples should give pause to critics who reject the community development model simply because it lacks the appearance of traditional social services or neighborhood activism. I conclude by drawing out lessons for students of community work.

IMAGES OF SUCCESS

By 1991, community-based development organizations had completed more than 320,000 units of housing for poor people, brought on line more than 17.4 million square feet of commercial or industrial space, and created or saved 90,000 permanent jobs (National Congress for Community Economic Development, 1991a, p. 2). A 1995 update showed an additional 80,000 units of affordable housing built, 6.6 million more square feet of commercial or industrial space provided, as well as $200,000,000 lent to businesses within poor communities (National Congress for Community Economic Development, 1995). CBDOs are central to the entire affordable housing industry, having produced 15.7% of all federally assisted affordable housing in the last 30 years (Center for Public Finance and Housing, 1994, p. 21).

On my site visits, I examined a wide variety of development projects: homeowners are helped to refurbish deteriorated properties; affordable, modern town homes are built replacing burnt out hulks; or a convent, too expensive for the archdiocese to maintain, is reconstructed as affordable housing for the community elderly. A CBDO recycles an abandoned car dealership into a community owned auto-repair and body shop, while a closed-down neighborhood school is converted into a care facility for the Medicaid elderly. In partnership with chain supermarkets, CBDOs open stores to provide affordable, quality food and household goods in neighborhoods that have no supermarkets, causing grocery bills to drop 38% (Sullivan, 1993, p. 125), while assuring that community members are employed in the store and that the product lines match ethnic expectations.

In an ethnically mixed neighborhood, an abandoned supermarket is turned into a Mercado, providing space for low-income people to sell needed goods. Another CBDO constructs a plaza containing a few stores and the neighborhood's first public library, while using the second story for affordable apartments. An abandoned facility for repairing railroad cars is transformed into a factory in which the formerly unemployed work to repair industrial palettes.

Transitional facilities are built for the homeless. Families are enabled to move out of squalid, public housing into their own homes, made affordable through sweat equity contributions and deep subsidies obtained by the development organizations. Middle class individuals–police officers, fire fighters, and tradesmen–pillars of neighborhood solidarity, are lured back into the inner city by the availability of affordable homes built by CBDOs (Rubin, 1993a; 1993b; 1995a).

As nonprofits with the skills of commercial developers, CBDOs combine resources from foundations and government along with those of the private sector. CBDOs approach commercial investors, banks, and for-profit partners, spread sheet in hand, showing that investors can make money in community projects. Simultaneously, the CBDO solicits from government, foundations, and churches the subsidy needed to keep property affordable. Then developmental organizations work with social agencies to help potential tenants or future owners overcome problems of debt, drugs, or dysfunctional families. Unlike for-profit capitalist developers, community-based development organizations intentionally seek risky endeavors on the hope that these projects will catalyze further community renewal.

QUESTIONING SUCCESS

Some projects seem to please community developers, social service providers, and advocates alike. In one central city, a community-based development organization refurbished a derelict apartment building to house handicapped individuals and their care givers. The project provided a vital social service, accomplished the goals of the activist neighborhood association of repairing a derelict building, and, through clever funding, earned enough money to contribute positively to the bottom line of the CBDO. More often, development deals necessitate a delicate balance between being financially viable, providing a social service, and encouraging efforts at community empowerment.

The Double Bottom Line

As social service scholars point out, CBDOs must balance out a bottom line between providing economically viable commercial projects or housing, or helping community members and clients overcome social problems. The reality is that many clients of CBDOs face profound personal problems and the neighborhoods in which CBDOs work confront arson, drugs, and economic and social deterioration. The tension between social obligation and financial wherewithal has been termed the " 'double bottom line'— the simultaneous need for *financial accountability* and attention to the nonprofit organization's *social goals* . . . many nonprofit housing sponsors have had to struggle mightily with this duality, given the inexorable logic of 'the numbers' " (Bratt, Keyes, Schwartz, & Vidal, 1994, p. 3).

Studies show that when projects are financially marginal, CBDOs pay less attention to social services and more to keeping the project afloat (Bratt, Keyes, Schwartz, & Vidal, 1994; Hebert, Heintz, Chris, & Wallace, 1993). Activists argue that concerns with economic viability distort a social mission. As one leader in the field explained, for a economically viable CBDO "managing success is the most difficult task you can do. . . . You've got all these assets. And all of a sudden–you are like a dog chasing a car–you caught the car now you are part of the traffic problem."

Success creates commitments to maintain a technical staff or grant writers whose salaries must be met. Or success might cause a CBDO to provide a social service at a loss and then face up to the longer-run financial implications. A development leader explained the tradeoffs in running a subsidized day-care center:

> [I]t's really a hard balance . . . The day center . . . and the services it's providing, it's terrific. . . . We're serving a tremendous amount of kids. And we're losing about $100,000 a year . . . we'd accumulated enough money over the years that we can subsidize this for a period of time but you reach a point where you have to make a decision that "Hey, that's it."

Or, as another example, when acting as landlords, CBDO directors are torn on whether to let an impoverished tenant's delinquent rent ride for a month or two. Owners explain:

> We have to collect the rent. We're not a social service agency . . . but in dealing with people [we] realize that there are a lot

of folks who live in our units that have multiple problems. We've got babies having babies. . . . We've got people with very low education levels, people who are getting AFDC and towards the end of the month the food stamps run out so that's what I mean, just to empathize, to realize that people have these problems.

This individual was torn, but reluctantly concluded "if people can't pay the rent they still have to go." Other studies, though, report that CBDOs "sometimes 'let the heart overrule the head' and in a compassionate effort not to evict delinquent tenants neglect to collect rents" (Sullivan, 1993, p. 28).

In another example of the tension between heart and head, a developmental activist described a project to build housing for displaced women and provide these women with a supportive social network. She was warned by her mentor that "You'd better . . . get yourself to an understanding: Do you want to develop housing or do you want to take care of people, you can't do both." She appreciated what was said, yet felt ambivalent: "Hearing the advice, was real sobering, it was very good to hear that because the reality is no you can't. *But I'm still believing that there is a way.*" She continued in her efforts to do both, thereby complicating getting the funding and delaying completion of the housing by an extra year.

The balance between the bottom line and the obligation to help people is compounded by pressure from funders who argue that CBDOs should ignore social service issues and concentrate on building numerous homes and creating their own asset base (Giloth, Orlebeke, Tickell, & Wright, 1992; National Congress for Community Economic Development, 1991b; Rubin, 1995a). For instance, in Cleveland, the guiding plan of the major funder was entitled "Pathways to Production," a policy blueprint that encouraged CBDOs to create their own assets by "producing to scale." Government, banks, and even foundations demand that CBDOs support themselves, in part, from overhead profits from the homes, yet to do so while also providing social services is an impossibility (Rubin, 1995b).

Some community-based development organizations concede to these pressures and focus mainly on their bottom line. Yet, to condemn the development model because of such capitulations would be equivalent to rejecting direct action advocacy just because many protest efforts are defeated (Rubin & Rubin, 1992; Woliver, 1993).

Abandoning Organizing for Development

A second criticism of CBDOs is that the focus on development weakens neighborhood advocacy efforts (Marquez, 1993, Stoecker, 1995). Is it possible for a CBDO to join in advocacy work when its leaders must interact with the very bankers and political officials against whom activists protest? Polemicists warn community developers that "ignoring their roots in political protest and organizing . . . puts them on a collision course with their poor constituents" (Lenz, 1988, p. 24).

Such tensions are recognized within the CBDO movement, though seen more as a pragmatic issue than one of philosophy: "Organizing, well if I don't go out and talk to these people, today, I can talk to them next week. But, if I don't get this [financial] stuff in line for the development, it's not going to happen."

Another fear is that CBDOs with their independent financial base can dominate neighborhood associations that are often financially impecunious. Activist-scholars suggest that neighborhood associations with a democratically elected membership should set an agenda for development that is then carried out by the CBDO as a technical arm of the neighborhood association (Stoecker, 1993; Medoff & Sklar, 1994). A study of the Dudley Street Neighborhood Initiative shows that such a model is possible (Medoff & Sklar, 1994). Yet, other scholars question if having neighborhood organizations control development is truly equivalent to democratic empowerment. Goetz and Sidney, for instance, argue almost the opposite.

> Research shows that neighborhood organizations are likely to be dominated by . . . residents with higher incomes. . . . On the other hand, [CBDOs] have led efforts to assist low-income residents . . . when neighborhood groups are captured by conservative property owners. . . . Thus, the suggestion that

[CBDOs] are less oppositional than voluntary neighborhood associations is not supported by the evidence. (Goetz & Sidney, 1995, p. 17)

MODEL FOR EMPOWERED COMMUNITY-BASED DEVELOPMENT

My conversational partners described models of how to balance doing development with the advocacy and social service activities needed to create an empowered community. To these developmental activists, providing services or doing deals is not an either/or proposition; rather each approach is accomplished within a holistic model of community renewal. In addition, while they recognize that CBDOs are not a substitute for traditional advocacy work, developmental activists actively lobby and protest. The goal of all three approaches–development, services, and advocacy–is to enable the poor and poor communities to gain a material stake in the nation's wealth.

Holistic Development: Combining Social Services and Physical Redevelopment

Community-based development organizations are involved in social services. The Urban Institute reports that about half of the CBDOs provide homeowners' or tenants' counseling, 28% do job training, while only 10% are exclusively physical developers (Center for Public Finance and Housing, 1994, pp. 55-56). Mercer Sullivan's anthropological investigations document numerous ways developmental activists provide social services within their housing projects, from counselling to family services (Sullivan, 1993).

Developmental activists argue that physical development is a means and not the end toward broader community renewal efforts and that their work is about helping people and neighborhoods through creating economic empowerment. A national leader rhetorically asked what would the logic be of building "condominiums in a neighborhood where people don't have jobs" while describing why CBDOs work on housing, job creation, and employment training simultaneously.

Revolving loan funds, in which start-up capital is lent to micro-entrepreneurs, most often women or minority group members, accomplish social ends that to developmental activists are as important as the economic goals. A director of a revolving loan fund argued "you pay as much attention to developing the business owner as you are paying to the developing the business, that you can't separate the two out from another." In such programs, people learn about spread sheets and the bottom line, but also participate in self-improvement efforts that "erase those negative messages and replace them with messages that say 'I can do this; it's time for me to do this; I deserve to be able to do this.'" Sweat equity programs in which home owners, in lieu of a down payment, commit themselves to hundreds of hours of work to repair the very buildings they will own have social as well as economic effects. Sweat equity builds in a psychological ownership to the property since the owner has contributed to its physical repair.

Doing economic development is about enabling community businesses to expand their supportive networks; it is as much about empowerment through having the opportunities, as it is a financial transaction. A CBDO director portrayed the blur between the social and economic role of his organization as it worked with a community business:

> The place I go to lunch . . . He's got a Mexican restaurant, he is starting to catch on. . . . we . . . loan him a $1,000 to buy a new refrigeration system. And, he begins to pay us back and . . . we expand it to $5,000 so he can do some remodeling. . . . All the while what we are doing is help him build a credit history. And, then we are working with a bank that . . . has agreed to buy any loan that is performing out of our portfolio. . . . The idea here is not to make [the community entrepreneur] a permanent client of [the CBDO] but to serve as the bridge to get into banking relationship.

Similarly, social services are necessitated by the very effort of a CBDO to maintain its property. But then the services take on a life and value of their own. A housing developer described that,

We sort of waded into the social service area. . . . Two years ago we said "jeez we've got all of these kids during the summer, what are they going to do." And, we need to provide them with some structured activities so they are not raising hell and destroying the property. . . . So we said, "let's put together a summer program . . . and we'll do a little remedial education and activities." So we started out with a summer program. . . . And . . . [it] became more of an academic enrichment program [run within the housing].

Lease purchase home ownership programs, programs in which poor people co-own housing with a CBDO and in which rental payments are treated as part of down payment, are often tied to social service activities. To assure that the tenants will eventually be able to assume title, the CBDOs sponsor programs to teach their co-owners about budgeting and preventative maintenance, skills necessary for the future homeowners (Cassidy, n.d.).

To maintain property, CBDOs set up rather stringent rules for tenants and future owners. For example, developmental activists are well aware of the social pressures on poor families to share space with friends and relatives, but recognize that such sharing creates overcrowding and rapid deterioration of the housing. Rules against space sharing protect both the CBDO and the newly housed tenant. As a development activist explained,

When we give someone a [lease-purchase] house that's probably the best house that they ever lived [in] . . . then they have something to protect and when we set down the rules [that] anybody who . . . stays with you more than 48 hours has to go on the lease. Then they've got a definable set of parameters to share with people who would otherwise want to come in and be part of their good fortune.

Community-based development organizations end up working closely with the social agencies that serve the people that CBDOs house, sometimes through the social service networks to which CBDOs are linked. Often the goal is to bring together both those in need and the support agencies. A CBDO director described a mixed use building that his organization had rehabilitated. The building contained commercial space on the street floor and apartments above for the homeless, and was attached to another structure in which the CBDO housed substance-dependent women:

> [We] . . . lease to nonprofit organizations that are providing services . . . the Salvation Army leases a space from us for [a] homeless assistance reception center. There's a drop-in center . . . it's kind of the living room for the SRO . . . here's a . . . clinic which is free health care for the homeless or people in the area. . . . We have the AIDS Resource Center located in our building too.

Through renting out such space, the CBDO became the node of an emerging network of community social service providers, and later was instrumental in forming a neighborhood social services coalition.

Projects are chosen that cost the CBDO funds, but that respond to social needs within the community. CBDOs work with tenants in crime patrols within their neighborhoods, subsidizing in part, training programs. Bethel, in Chicago, has run aggressive campaigns to attack the drug trade, both by holding prayer vigils outside of drug distribution centers and with direct action marches to the suburbs from which the purchasers of the drugs come. The housing director of a major CBDO described why her organization repaired a derelict building that was far more expensive to fix than were other available sites. The complex had been the center of drug trade for the south side of the city and the CBDO "recognize[d] that the whole adjacent block was so much of a threat that nobody in the world was going to want to buy a house knowing that they are next to a crime infested [building]."

Other CBDOs integrate social services into holistic strategies. Elsewhere, I detail how a CBDO linked a program to rebuild homes to a community effort to teach teenagers construction skills. It then used these homes as sites for a home-day care service that was owned by former AFDC clients, who the CBDO, in turn, helped gain certification (Rubin, 1994). In a similar vein, Bethel set up social service agencies in buildings physically developed by the CBDO and then taught community members to become service providers (Barry, 1989). The New Communities Corporation in

Newark (NCC), the nation's best-known CBDO, has built day care centers that care for children of those involved in job training programs, and provides job training programs for the formerly homeless now housed in buildings owned by NCC for possible placement in businesses set up by the CBDO.

Economic development projects blur into social service work benefiting the overall community. Through a direct action campaign, a community-based development organization got possession of an abandoned auto repair training center that was then used to provide job training in the auto repair and related businesses. More than 150 individuals, mostly Hispanic, have graduated from the auto repair program and obtained jobs in for-profit dealerships, while other neighborhood businesses have been spun off from the initial enterprise, including a welding and metal bending business, auto salvage and parts recycling enterprise, as well as a day-care center and an asbestos removal service.

This economic development program had important social consequences for community members, as the organization

> find[s] people who nobody wants who have incredible talents . . . Our tow truck driver . . . came in here three years ago under the welfare . . . he knows every car we got in our lot. . . . He knows which fender is good shape, which isn't . . . he is in charge of our reclamation project. . . . He is a diamond. And, yet, the system had him as useless.

This development activist continued by describing the community mission accomplished by the economic development projects:

> People who come from Mexico or Puerto Rico they gravitate here. . . . Everybody speaks Spanish. . . . You know, some of our mechanics have been people who didn't speak English, but were crack mechanics. . . . They were on welfare; no one would hire them; they couldn't speak English. We put them to work for $12 an hour.

Learning business skills in a supportive environment empowers community members. People are able to form their own enterprises as the CBDO can buffer them during periods of low business or equipment failure. For instance, a CBDO helped a community member, Freddy, move from unemployment to ownership of his own asbestos removal service. Early on, Freddy's new business faced a major problem with damaged equipment that could have bankrupted his start-up firm. The CBDO stepped in and repaired the equipment on credit, until this community firm was more financially stable. In this case the goal of the CBDO was to help community members overcome the disadvantages society has placed on them because they are poor and minority.

> [I]f you want community people to get in business you're going to have give them an edge because right now the playing field is dominated by capital. . . . If Freddy had started off with his asbestos business by himself 2 years ago he'd probably be dead about now. . . . Now he knows how to run the business and he's going to have a real good chance of not only surviving but of expanding and growing and being a real vital business in the community because he had the opportunity under our umbrella.

Economic development projects stimulated by the CBDO bring in wealth to the broader neighborhood. In addition, these projects have social spillovers for the young, through the presence of role models.

> Even now [as] Freddy's spinning off his business . . . younger people . . . see that he's going to run a business. They know him as a community person. We could bring in a [downtown] business man and say look "he's going to mentor you" but he doesn't look like 'em, he doesn't dress like 'em, he doesn't eat like 'em, he doesn't smell like 'em nothing and so they think "well that's nice he's a business man but I could never be that." But with the people that we have here as role models then the youth who come into our programs . . . get the idea that, "hey if they could do it I could do it."

Finally, as those helped by the CBDO gain a financial stake in the neighborhood the community is empowered. The developmental activist, a former voter rights worker, explained how having a good job creates political empowerment:

[Voting] didn't come by getting them at meetings and telling how important voting is. It came by them starting to have some economic independence. Jose, our general manager never voted before in his life. . . . He just bought a house and he had a job. He said "I want to vote for that Hispanic guy." Something I couldn't get him to do for fifteen years. He says, "I got a house now, I got a car, I got a job. And, my kids, you know, are in the school."

Hey. That's social change you know. It didn't happen by having voter registration drives. It happened by giving people a stake economically and then they turn on.

With holistic economic development, the CBDO plays a far bigger role than that of builder or financier. The wealth provided by the development organization becomes the base for both social and political empowerment.

Advocacy as Part of the Development Model

Needing public funding, community-based development organizations are cautious about engaging in direct actions. As one leader described, "You should never bite the hand that feeds but if you know you got to bite that hand, you shouldn't go to them for food." But then, somewhat contradictorily, he detailed a year-long direct action campaign his organization spearheaded against the city government.

Yet, to a surprising degree, development organizations are involved in advocacy efforts to empower themselves, the people with whom they work, and the broader communities in which they are located. The Urban Institute reports that two-thirds of CBDOs do community organizing, about half provide homeowners' or tenants' counseling, and a third do advocacy to support the Community Reinvestment Act, the law that pressures banks to reinvest in communities of the poor (Center for Public Finance and Housing, 1994). Goetz and Sidney (1995, p. 5) report from Vidal (1992, p. 36) that many CBDOs are "an outgrowth of other ongoing community-based activities [including] opposition to urban renewal plans, Community Reinvestment Act challenges, tenant organizing . . ."

and cite Gittell, Gross and Newman's (1994) findings that "50 percent [of the CBDOs] engaged in community organizing and 25 percent did tenant organizing" (Goetz and Sidney, 1995, p. 5). Further, even when successful at development, CBDOs do not drift away from activism as "there was just as much organizing activity among the older [CBDOs] as among recently-formed [CBDOs], suggesting that these groups are not less likely to organize residents as they grow" (Goetz & Sidney, 1995, p. 6).

Community-based development organizations are involved in advocacy work both to gain resources they need for development as well as to support broader community change (Goetz & Sidney, 1995, p. 4). In many impoverished communities, the CBDO is the only institution that can provide a base for collective action. As an example, when Bethel began its development work in the west side of Chicago, there simply were no other organizations in its neighborhood doing either advocacy or development, so the CBDO had to do both.

By their very effort to build homes to house the poor and minorities, CBDOs end up as advocates for progressive change in opposition to conservative neighborhood associations. Goetz and Sidney (1994) detail how a neighborhood association was so angered at the progressive work of the CBDO that it destroyed the CBDO because the development agency was the social advocate in the neighborhood. The CBDO provided affordable housing for minorities, thereby changing the racial composition of the community, while working with tenants in privately owned buildings to organize against unresponsive landlords, all the while promoting tenant self-management in the buildings owned by the CBDO itself. The CBDO's advocating for and with the poor was too much for the homeowner-dominated neighborhood association to tolerate.

In doing advocacy, community-based development organizations follow two approaches. The first parallels the conventional neighborhood advocacy model in which community members forcefully attack institutions, disinvesting from the community. With the second approach, one that I term the new advocacy, CBDOs form coalitions of development groups that in turn create meta-coalitions of progressive organizations to lobby and advocate for resources to rebuild neighborhoods of the poor.

Advocating for Development Within the Neighborhoods

CBDOs, in alliances with churches and community associations, engage in direct actions that pressure banks to live up to their Community Reinvestment Act obligations and encourage cities to keep promises made to the poor. In one case, the CBDO was asked by other community organizations to help save a hospital that was about to close. The tactics used were reminiscent of the civil rights era:

> One of the big mobilizing things was . . . a pray-vigil around the hospital . . . [we] got twenty churches out, and got enough folks out to have a hand to hand around the whole square block of the hospital with candles. And, then once we made the whole human link around the hospital and prayed. . . .
>
> But that was a wonderful mobilizing event, the hospital staff saw that people really cared. . . . And, then the leaders met and made the pitch to the mother organization, corporate head-quarters, and said "okay, here is what we have done. Now you have to commit to us that you are going to leave this hospital open for a year."

Most CBDO-inspired protests, though, are targeted at banks that are reluctant to live up to their Community Reinvestment Act responsibilities. A development activist shared his experiences when a bank was withdrawing capital from the community:

> The bank wasn't happy. . . . We showed them all these data and statistics . . . about twenty churches [came] along with us . . . "we want to sit down and put a program together." And, the bank declined. . . .
>
> And . . . what we had to do was bring out the peoples.
>
> And, we brought bus loads of people into the bank lobby, into the streets, around the bank. We had churches call up. . . . The bank couldn't communicate to business for three days.
>
> The bank was developing a new bank. . . . We sent bus loads of people over there to stop the contractors. The contractors couldn't do any work. So we just shut down the whole operation.

> We said, "you don't want to talk with us poor people with a legitimate plan. We don't come to fight, we come to talk." The bank wasn't used to sitting down and talking with poor, low income people . . . we were organized, and we pulled the churches in and the community was in. And we shut the bank down for a few days. . . .

This protest and other similar ones encouraged banks in that city to negotiate a city-wide community reinvestment package to be run under the supervision of a board that contained community activists.

Other action campaigns forcefully remind government of its obligations in poor communities. An activist described how her CBDO led a coalition of churches to city hall to argue with the mayor for support in an affordable housing program. The threat of direct action was present as each of these churches could bring out people, and on other occasions had done so. She paraphrased the argument made to the mayor:

> These twenty churches want you to become a partner and this is what we need from you. One we need free land. You are biggest holder, you are the biggest slumlord in our community. What better way of getting land back upon the tax roll . . . there are a number of [ways] . . . you can help us lower the cost of the home. One, you charge for building permit. We want that fee waived. . . . Two, we wanted water and sewer tap fee and inspection waived [and that] . . . is going to be passed on to the borrower in terms of savings.

Protest tactics are used in this case and in others, but the demands are for the wherewithal to permit a sophisticated development organization to carry out a project that benefits the community.

In another case, a community-based development organization wanted to refurbish an abandoned school building to provide office space for community services, but

> The city manager did not see the city . . . as providing social services in the community. . . . The community then stood in arms. We came down in mass, a hundred people and they

picked three or four people to testify on behalf of the community and behalf of the neighborhood. . . . The . . . city council
agreed with the community and not the city manager.

CBDOs also pay the salary of street-level community organizers
who work within the neighborhoods. By helping neighborhoods
organize, the CBDO gains support for doing its projects, but in turn
the CBDO discovers that the projects must be those approved by the
broader community.

A community developer narrated how the organizer, Gladys,
hired by his CBDO, worked with the neighborhood in defining and
then gaining support for a plan to replace a derelict block of businesses. Initially, the CBDO wanted to replace businesses with an
updated commercial area, but changed its goal to affordable housing to respond to community concerns:

> The commercial strip was a terrible, very, very blighted two-
> block neighborhood that . . . hosted a major portion of the
> city's illegal drug activity, prostitution, crime in general, ille-
> gal liquor sale. . . .
> Now the commercial strip [ownership] is almost all black,
> 99% black and we need black and white folks to thrash this
> [project] out. . . . So Gladys essentially organized people . . .
> we had as many as 200 people at these meetings and people
> were mad, people were excited, people were pessimistic said it
> would never happen. . . . Someone said to tear this down to get
> rid of the drug dealers; other people said you are tearing this
> down so rich white folk could move in.
> People who ran these businesses employed big-time attor-
> neys; they had all kinds of solid, workable, manageable, politi-
> cal connections. And, here came along a scrappy, neighbor-
> hood people who said it is over. "We think, these strips are a
> blight on the neighborhood, we got to get rid of them." . . .
> And the neighborhood said "what we want in its place is
> affordable housing." . . . Then people look to us and say, you
> are a developer, let [the CBDO] do the affordable housing
> because we know who will manage it. . . .
> Gladys helps us organize that . . . neighborhood people
> don't trust any institution. None. None. None. None. Black

> neighborhood people don't trust white people unless they known them a long time. . . . Gladys grew up right back here . . . everybody knows her. I am from this community too. . . . All our staff lives in the neighborhood. So we are available, we are vulnerable and that makes a big difference.

As the CBDO worked to gain support for the project through organizing efforts, the community itself was empowered to guide the agenda for the development organization.

The New Advocacy:
Working with Coalitions and Support Structure

Funding for community development work depends in large part upon governmental programs, the low-income housing tax credit, the community development block grant, and a variety of state, national, and local housing subsidies. Much of the support from government is a result of legislative lobbying and broad scale advocacy efforts, many of them led by coalitions of community-based development organizations and traditional advocacy organizations.

Such protests use the Community Reinvestment Act as a wedge to force banks to set up loan pools for reinvestment in communities of the poor. These pools are often monitored by developmental activists from CBDOs whose participation assures that a battle initially won through pressure and lobbying is not lost later on in the implementation stage, through lack of technical knowledge (Rubin & Rubin, 1992, p. 450). One such activist described:

> I sit on the reinvestment board of [four banks]. . . . And . . . the economic development board of the city. . . . I watches all the money to make sure the underserved communities get their fair share. . . . I know better . . . than those guys with those fancy ties and shirts on. . . . I don't back up. . . . They are not used to having community people pull the bullet. . . . Because I get the statistics. . . . I got time for that because it is empowering the black community, the poor community, the community that no banks is going to deal with.

On the national level mixed coalitions build up from a disparate collection of organizations including the Local Initiative Support

Corporation, a funder; the National Congress for Community Economic Development, the trade association for community-based development organizations; and the activist Center for Community Change, along with other advocates for affordable housing which convinced Congress to make permanent the Low Income Housing Tax Credit, a principal source of money for affordable housing. Goetz (1992, 1993) describes how city-wide housing coalitions with CBDOs as members conduct activist campaigns to pressure local governments to expand investment in affordable housing or to set up Housing Trust Funds, dedicated streams of money for affordable housing.

In Massachusetts, the state legislature was persuaded to fund development organizations by a direct action/lobbying campaign led by the trade association for community developers. In Ohio, coalitions of community-based development organizations joined together with housing advocacy organizations in a successful campaign to convince both the legislature and the citizenry to approve a constitutional amendment making housing a public purpose.

In Chicago, the REHAB Network, a coalition of housing developers, pressured the city government to redirect hundreds of millions into community-based projects. This effort involved direct one-on-one lobbying and Alinsky-style protests in a campaign "which includes over 260 neighborhood developers, community organizations, churches and advocacy organizations" (Chicago Rehab Network, 1994). The decision to do advocacy emerged during a coalition-sponsored workshop in which the developers lamented how they had become too passive because of their fear of losing funding. The coalition asked a university research center to analyze statistics about housing needs, and with this information, contracted with an Alinsky-style organizer to coordinate a non-violent, direct-action campaign that pressured city politicians to reinvest hundreds of millions in disadvantaged neighborhoods (Ervin, 1994).

By undertaking advocacy as part of a coalition, community-based development organizations handle the tension between doing pressureful actions and the fear of retribution from those in power. A coalition director explained,

> My board president [a head of a CBDO] will not go to the
> mayor's office . . . and say "look God damn it you better put
> some more money into housing right now or we are going to
> call a press conference blasting the fact that city did less than a
> 100 units of housing last year." But he will call me up and say
> "you get your butt over there and do it." . . . My board
> president has a three million dollar deal sitting there for the
> mayor to sign off on.

Tactics followed by coalitions of CBDOs follow the entire pano-
ply of those described in organizing texts, varying from straightfor-
ward lobbying to sit-ins. For instance, NCCED successfully spearheaded a national lobbying effort for Congress to set aside money
for community development organizations; in Illinois, a statewide
developers association working with an advocacy organization
massed its membership and with one-on-one confrontations pressured the legislature, and overcame the opposition of the real estate
industry, to set up a housing transfer fee to pay for an Affordable
Housing Fund. In another state, when funding for affordable housing was threatened, the state coalition set up the

> first annual neighborhood fax-in . . . community organizing
> for the 90's. We found out that there were two fax machines in
> the [state] house; two in the Senate and one in the governor's
> office. And we inundated those SOB's.

Other tactics included intimidating the opposition through the
threat of disclosing embarrassing background facts. For instance,
CANDO, another coalition of CBDOs in Chicago, pressured the
city into using unspent federal grant money for neighborhood projects by threatening to leak how slowly the city was drawing down
funds available from HUD. Here the threat worked since the Mayor
had been publicly claiming concern for the neighborhoods and after
privately capitulating to the pressure took credit himself for CAN-
DO's proposal.

On another occasion, a meta-coalition of coalitions of CBDOs
and neighborhood associations campaigned to force the city to redirect its capital budget away from downtown. Through background
data analysis, this coalition learned that all city wards except the

downtown were dramatically underserved on capital projects. Next, using this data, members of the coalition convinced the aldermen (sic) in their wards that the neighborhoods they represented were being deprived of needed projects. The meta-coalition then held a sit-in at city hall to give the aldermen the political screen vis-à-vis the mayor to insist on a more equitable distribution of capital projects.

Elsewhere, governmental officials have worked behind the scenes with advocacy organizations and CBDOs to pressure banks to set up community reinvestment pools. A ranking governmental official described to me that while he was conducting negotiations with the banks to improve community reinvestment, he encouraged people in the community movement to picket the bank's president's house. In the same state, the director of the CBDO association organized mass meetings in individual legislative districts to pressure legislators to support housing done by nonprofits. She described the pressure tactics at the "large community meetings where you have a hundred people from your neighborhood" who talk to officials about the benefits from community development projects. Such meetings are a "very empowering thing for people. . . . it gets people out to vote because they feel that they can have a direct relationship and a direct impact on how government affects their lives."

The new advocacy can be effective in persuading government and banks to support progressive community change. Moreover, in forming the coalitions such efforts bring together both physical developers and traditional neighborhood activists in situations in which each can learn from the other.

Guiding Carpentry with a Social Conscience

To explain why they do what they do, leading developmental activists have worked out an organic theory that links their efforts to broader traditions of community work. An organic theory is formulated as those working to bring about social change reflect upon their experiences and interpret what these experiences mean and what actions they imply (cf. Rubin, 1994 for more detail). Organic theories emerge through the contestation and confrontation of daily activity (Lipsitz, 1988) and offer "guidelines in working through the dilemmas [activists] confront" (Posner, 1990, p. 5). The content of organic theories is shared in discussions at workshops, retreats, conventions, special seminars, and through reflective writings, as well as in the interviews given to sociologists such as myself.

I will briefly sketch the five linked components of the organic theory described to me by the community developers (for more detail see Rubin, 1993a; 1993b; 1994; 1995a):

- Developers have a moral obligation through their work to symbolize hope for those in poor communities
- Empowerment occurs by encouraging both material ownership and the acceptance of social responsibilities
- Renewal involves building an economically autarchic community
- To provide hope, empowerment, and build economic autarchy, requires a holistic strategy, uniting development with social services, while not shunning advocacy
- To bring about a holistic strategy CBDOs act as niche organizations that stimulate and coordinate others

The initial premise of this organic theory is that community developers have a moral obligation to begin the process of renewal, for instance by tackling the most difficult projects to demonstrate the possibility of change. The underlying philosophy was expressed as "*I mean if we don't do it, nobody's going to do it.*" The moral obligation is to battle poverty as an example to stimulate others to join in the battle. One individual expressed this as:

> We think of ourselves as catalysts . . . we've done over 600 units of housing. . . . But the fact of the matter is, it is a drop in a bucket. So if that drop doesn't . . . ignite activism and ignite a sense among people about what can be done when people work collectively and struggle for what is needed, then we've done little.

To 'ignite others' the CBDO shows the possibility for change, for example by taking "on the worst of the worst of the worst and pave the way for the guys who want to make some money."

The moral obligation is to show there is hope for improvement, by making successes quite prominent:

> We like to focus on a lot of things that are as visible as possible. . . . new housing is much more visible, a shot in the arm, something that people can rally around. . . . It gives people a sense of ownership in the non-traditional, non-capitalistic sense.

Ownership both in a material and a psychological sense is empowering. A developer explained how even rental housing empowers, since in the project described

> the tenants will be involved in making key decisions affecting their own housing. They will decide who will be renting the unit next door, they will be deciding what are the rules about storing broken down cars. . . . We are giving . . . the renter . . . a sense of ownership; we're giving them a stake. We're letting them see how their actions or failure to act . . . has impact upon the housing.

What the organic theory implies is that to create empowerment requires people to have ownership of material things, as well as owning psychologically a better sense of self. Ownership gives people a material stake in the society and is thereby empowering, for instance in the satisfaction felt when poor people end up moving from welfare to owning their own business. And, empowerment occurs as people who have been excluded learn that their efforts pay off in material advantages for themselves and their communities.

One of the most memorable moments of this study occurred as an elderly woman, a tenant in a housing complex for the elderly built by a community development organization, addressed an assembled group of developmental activists. She described her pride of being able to speak in front of a large group, a skill taught her by the CBDO. Then she detailed how she worked to organize elderly people in a successful campaign to pressure government to fund construction of a nursing home adjacent to the housing complex. While the CBDO would hold title to the nursing home, the elderly residents had psychic ownership and the security that when they needed care they did not have to move away from their friends.

The organic theory continues: home ownership or having a material stake in society in general creates empowerment through rooting people within a geographic place and social structure. Listen to this exchange between myself and an organic theorist about the linkage between having things and being rooted:

> *Activist:*   What is it that made you successful? . . . You own things. . . . You own stuff. What do you own? Tell me what you own.
>
> *HJR:*   Me, personally? Home, couple cars, hefty retirement funds. . . . Computer. . . .
>
> *Activist:*   Got a wife?
>
> *HJR:*   Yeah. I don't own her.
>
> *Activist:*   Let's talk about it in the possessive. . . . You have mothers and fathers and brothers. *But you own the problem. But it keeps you linked somehow to all this stuff.* History, memory, all kinds of things that you own, through the psychic as well as material. You own all kinds of stuff. . . . What does the 'beneath the underclass' own? . . . They own nothing. How do you begin to develop ownership? . . . Well, you give 'em the same thing that everybody's got.

He then argued that development work is about creating rootedness through the self-respect and responsibility created by material ownership.

Empowerment through ownership benefits the broader community through strategies to circulate wealth within neighborhoods of need. Efforts by CBDOs to weatherize homes or provide heat-efficient furnaces stop wealth from being exported to the utilities, wealth that can then be spent in the neighborhood. Opening a community enterprise, the Mercado for instance, or the auto-repair shop, keeps jobs within the community. The goal of a CBDO becomes that of targeting job and employment programs that recycle money inside the community, not simply introducing funds to the community that then are spent elsewhere.

Several CBDOs extended the idea of empowerment through individual ownership to a broader sense of community control. These CBDOs worked with people to help them own homes, often through sweat equity programs. But then rather than totally privatizing the new wealth, the CBDO shared both the responsibility and benefits of the wealth with the wider community. One way of doing so was through community land trusts in which a representative community body maintained title to land underlying the new homes. Doing so assured that the overall community could be certain that when homes were sold by their initial owners, prices could be kept reasonable, allowing other poor people to benefit from the same properties.

Empowering people who have started out in one-down positions requires a holistic approach that unites development work with the provision of social services. One developer explained this logic of holistic development with her CBDO's welfare mothers program:

> Our problem was twofold. One is, to help women get off of welfare, you need day care. And, so we negotiated with the state . . . to pay for day care. . . . Then you come to find out that there . . . isn't enough day care here . . . [so we decide] let's train welfare mothers to become day care home providers, be self-employed . . . we then . . . train[ed] women in our community. And, come to find out that they cannot get licensed unless they are doing day care in the licensable space. And, most of them were living in apartments that would not pass muster.
>
> So we said well why don't we combine that with our self-help housing and let them move into brand new houses. Well here you have a welfare woman who is going to be self-employed, well how do you get a mortgage for her. . . . So we had to figure out, how could we do this.

She explained a complicated scheme for enabling the women to gain ownership in their homes that in turn would become the location for the day care service. Social services and physical redevelopment are joined together for holistic development.

Doing holistic projects such as day care efforts or bringing about the complicated training and job placement programs within the auto-repair shop necessitates that the community-based development organization coordinate a multitude of external resources. To accomplish such coordinative tasks, CBDOs become niche organizations by catalyzing others to join in and convincing the separate participants that their individual agendas will be accomplished in the broader project. For instance, to bring about the day care project required getting concurrent agreement between a local high school that provided training, the county welfare department, which handled the licensing for both child care and day-care homes, and 16 different funding sources.

Surviving in the niche means knowing when to cut a deal wearing a gray flannel suit and when to join with allies from the housing advocacy movement in more forceful actions. A CBDO can bridge the gap between advocates and the bankers by turning the results of a protest into a tangible project. As an example, protestors had unsuccessfully tried to stop a firm from abandoning one city, but as a sop from the city government received some promises of economic aid to the neighborhood. Little, though, occurred since the city had scant knowledge of how to bring about the needed development. A CBDO that had been part of the protest coalition stepped in and with the grateful support of the city, was able to get a federal development grant that allowed the CBDO, along with a for-profit partner, to build a commercial facility in the abandoned building. The space was then rented to firms that employed community members, including one large portion leased to another community-based development organization that moved a social service facility to the building–a facility that both provided services to those in the neighborhood and employed community members as service providers.

As a niche organization, a CBDO provides a place, sometimes literally a table, at which advocacy, social service, and governmental agencies can communicate about shared problems. A neighborhood chanced losing several hundred affordable apartments to upscale condominiums when a CBDO stepped in and coordinated the efforts of government, neighborhood organizations, social service groups, and an advocacy organization of the tenants to stop the harmful actions. The director of the CBDO described her role:

I got all these people around this table to care about the project as much as I did . . . by the end of the deal we'd built a team . . . Each of those people around the table was really, really critical to the deal. They each brought stuff that no one else brought, their expertise, their perspective. It was a real collaborative effort.

The CBDO's contribution then was to structure the financing and set up a non-profit corporation to own the building and maintain its affordability.

In another troubled neighborhood, several community social service agencies were at logger-heads. As a fiscally solvent organization, not dependent on the same funding as were the social service agencies, the CBDO offered a neutral table, at which agencies–social, governmental, and activist–could talk one with the another. The CBDO spoke the language of development, protest, and that of community empowerment through ownership. As such the CBDO

> is more and more functioning as a table where people come and sit around . . . because it's a safe table, with a stable group who's not trying to threaten people or take things on. We just want things to happen. And we're willing to put some money and staff to make it happen . . . and that's enabled a lot of conversations to begin happening.

The CBDO provided a physical place to meet and provided a forum for discussing issues of community change. And, according to the CBDO director, by doing so it is "creat(ing) an environment for the light bulbs to go off for other people in terms of the connections . . . housing is connected to jobs. Youth is connected to education."

LESSONS FOR COMMUNITY PRACTICE

I have presented an upbeat view of what community-based development organizations can and have accomplished. It is a portrait of possibility, yet one given credence by the number of homes already built and the jobs made available.

My work focuses upon successful organizations and does not analyze why other CBDOs have failed. Evidence exists of numerous failures: failures that occur because of lack of start-up funding, ill-conceived development projects, biting off too large a task, and occasional malfeasance. Most CBDOs are small, lack core funding, and can easily die before they bring about successful projects. Their production is often too low to generate the overhead that can maintain the core organization. Further, since community-based development organizations require public subventions to pay for the social overhead, organizations without a modest public support simply die (Bratt et al., 1994; Giloth et al., 1992; Vidal, 1989).

Another handicap facing the community development movement is the dearth of skilled developmental activists. These individuals need the patience and forbearance of community organizers with the business acumen of a free-booting, entrepreneurial capitalist. The only answer that I have to why individuals with combinations of such skills even work in the community development movement when they could earn far more as commercial developers is that they care for their neighborhoods and want to combat racial and gender injustices of which they as individuals have often been victim.

What lessons can students take from these successful CBDOs that can be applied to help other organizations renew hope among the poor?

First, community-based development must be seen as much as a set of attitudes and beliefs as it is a combination of technical skills. The goal of successful CBDOs is not simply to put up buildings, but to recreate a community, both in a physical and in a social-psychological sense. This perspective was shared by a director of a CBDO as he described why his organization undertook an economically risky condominium project: "you are concerned about what it does to the neighborhood . . . [the project] is not a money maker. That's not why we're doing it. *We're not home builders; we're community builders.*"

But even the most successful CBDOs realize that they cannot succeed unless they bring together diverse skills and resources. Within their neighborhoods, CBDOs unite social service, advocacy, and other development organizations. The work of developmental activists shows that mastering skills in social administration—in budgeting, personnel management, negotiations, in coordinating the work of multiple organizations, or preparing a spread sheet—need not imply withdrawal from a social change agenda. It is through skills in these technical matters that CBDOs are enabled to do the projects that renew hope and empower those within poor communities.

Another lesson students should note is that community organizations cannot work alone, but rather require help from one another. As I report in work in progress, CBDOs are part of a broadly structured, coordinated movement of organizations connected one to another through a cascading network of coalitions and trade associations. Doing development requires understanding how to build a coalition (Mizrahi & Rosenthal, 1993) and learning how to benefit from "community enabling structures" (Chavis, Florin, & Felix, 1993). The battle for change is a collective effort.

Further, developmental activists teach that values and ideological beliefs are not to be separated from action, and that abstract concepts have quite grounded meanings. In classes and texts in community work (my own included), the concept of "empowerment" is primarily treated as a psychological feeling. In contrast, the organic theorists within the community development movement argue that empowerment occurs both for their organizations and for individuals through the material ownership of goods, property, and social and job skills. Through such ownership individuals gain confidence to fight for more for themselves and for the broader community.

A final lesson that can be drawn is for students and scholars alike to tune down the shrill rhetoric that turns social service provider against direct action activist and both against the community developer. Rather the student should learn to think of the integration of different models for working with and helping communities in need.

Community-based development organizations are not about leading an in-the-streets revolution, but they are about increasing social equity. It is too easy to ignore this fact and complain that CBDOs have abandoned the fight for social change by building homes and seeking funding to do so. But it is equally easy to point out neighborhood associations that have failed from lack of community participation, or those that have been taken over by a small clique of self-centered individuals. Similarly, advocacy is about social change, but advocacy efforts often fail, are bought off, and even when seeming to prevail end up with no base for preserving what has been accomplished.

At their best, community-based development organizations demonstrate that physical development, social advocacy, and providing social services are not alternative choices, but rather complementary approaches to rebuild and restore communities. All three efforts–to build, to provide services, and to protest–merge as a responsive CBDO provides an empowered table around which other agencies can unite. Those advocating for social change and those teaching about community change would be well advised to learn from the CBDO model.

REFERENCES

Barry, P. (1989). *Rebuilding the walls: A nuts and bolts guide to the community development methods of Bethel New Life, Inc. in Chicago.* Chicago: Bethel New Life.

Berndt, H. (1977). *New rulers in the ghetto: The community development corporation and urban poverty.* Westport, CT: Greenwood Press.

Bratt, R. G., Keyes, L. C., Schwartz, A., & Vidal, A. C. (1994). *Confronting the management challenge: Affordable housing in the nonprofit sector.* New York: Community Development Research Center: Graduate School of Management and Urban Policy: New School for Social Research.

Cassidy, C. (n.d.). Lease-purchase: One road to home ownership. *Lessons of Enterprise, 1*(1), 1-12.

Center for Public Finance and Housing (1994). *Status and prospects of the nonprofit housing sector.* Washington, DC: Community and Economic Development Program, Urban Institute.

Chavis, D. M., Florin, P., Felix, M. (1993). Nurturing grassroots initiatives for community development: the role of enabling systems. In T. Mizrahi & J. D. Morrison (Eds.) *Community organization and social administration: Advances, trends and emerging principles* (pp. 41-68). New York: The Haworth Press, Inc.

Chicago Rehab Network (1994). "Victory" Chicago: Chicago Rehab Network.

Delgado, G. (1994). *Beyond the politics of place: New directions in community organizing in the 1990s.* Oakland, CA: Applied Research Center.

Ervin, M. (1994, February/March). Building blocks: a step-by-step organizing campaign leads to new funding for housing. *The Neighborhood Works, 17*(1), 10.

Giloth, R., Orlebeke, C., Tickell, J., & Wright, P. (1992). *Choices ahead: CDCs and real estate production in Chicago.* Chicago, IL: The Nathalie P. Vorhees Center for Neighborhood and Community Improvement.

Gittell, M., Gross, S. & Newman, K. (1994). Women and minorities in neighborhood development organizations. Paper presented at the Annual Meeting of the Urban Affairs Association, New Orleans, March 2-5.

Goetz, E. G. (1993). *Shelter burden: Local politics and progressive housing policy.* Philadelphia: Temple University Press.

Goetz, E. G. & Sidney, M. (1995). Community development corporations as neighborhood advocates: A study of the political activism of nonprofit developers. *Applied Behavioral Science Review, 3*(1), 1-20.

Goetz, E. G. & Sidney, M. (1994). Revenge of the property owners: Community development and the politics of property. *Journal of Urban Affairs, 16*(4), 319-334.

Goetz, E. G. (1992). Local government support for nonprofit housing: A survey of U.S. cities. *Urban Affairs Quarterly, 27*(3), 420-435.

Hebert, S., Heintz, K. B., Chris, K. N., & Wallace, J. E. (1993). *Non-profit housing: Costs and funding final report Volume I-Findings.* Abt Associates with Aspen Systems. Washington, DC.

Lenz, T. J. (1988, Spring). Neighborhood development: Issues and models. *Social Policy, 19*, 24-30.

Lipsitz, G. (1988). *A life in the struggle: Ivory Perry and the culture of opposition.* Philadelphia: Temple University Press.

Marquez, B. (1993, August). Mexican-American community development corporations and the limits of directed capitalism. *Economic Development Quarterly, 7*(3), 287-295.

Medoff, P., & Sklar, H. (1994). *Streets of hope: The fall and rise of an urban neighborhood.* Boston: South End Press.

Mizrahi, T., & Rosenthal, B. (1993). Managing dynamic tensions in social change coalitions. In T. Mizrahi & J. D. Morrison (Eds.) *Community organization and social administration: advances, trends and emerging principles* (pp. 11-40). New York: The Haworth Press, Inc.

National Congress for Community Economic Development. (1995). *Tying it all together: The comprehensive achievements of community-based development organizations.* Washington, DC: National Congress for Community Economic Development.

National Congress for Community Economic Development. (1991a). *Changing the Odds: The Achievements of Community-based Development Corporations.* Washington, DC: National Congress for Community Economic Development.

National Congress for Community Economic Development. (1991b). *Between and on Behalf: The Intermediary Role.* Washington, DC: National Congress for Community Economic Development.

Posner, P. (1990). Introduction. In J. Kling & P. Posner (Eds.), *Dilemmas of activism: Class, community, and the politics of local mobilization* (pp. 3-20). Philadelphia: Temple University Press.

Rubin, H. J. (1993a). Community empowerment within an alternative economy. In D. Peck & J. Murphy (Eds.), *Open institutions: The hope for democracy* (pp. 99-121). Westport, CT: Praeger.

Rubin, H. J. (1993b, September/October). Understanding the ethos of community-based development: Ethnographic description for public administration. *Public Administration Review, 53*(5), 428-437.

Rubin, H. J. (1994, August). There aren't going to be any bakeries here if there is no money to afford jellyrolls: The organic theory of community-based development. *Social Problems, 41*(4), 401-424.

Rubin, H. J. (1995a, May 1995). Renewing hope in the inner city: Conversations with community-based development practitioners. *Administration and Society*, 27(1), 127-160.

Rubin, H. J. (1995b, May). "Shoot the f . . . ing intermediaries, especially LISC": Theories of intermediation for community-based development. Paper Presented at the 25 Annual Meeting of the Urban Affairs Association. Portland, OR.

Rubin, H. J., & Rubin, I. S. (1995). *Qualitative interviewing: The art of hearing data*. Thousand Oaks, CA: Sage.

Rubin, H. J., & Rubin, I. S. (1992). *Community organizing and development* (second edition). Columbus, OH: Macmillan.

Stoecker, R. (1994). *Defending community: The struggle for alternative redevelopment in Cedar Riverside*. Philadelphia: Temple University Press.

Stoecker, R. (1995). Community, movement, organization: the problem of identity convergence in collective action. *The Sociological Quarterly*, 36(1), 111-130.

Sullivan, M. L. (1993). *More than housing: How community development corporations go about changing lives and neighborhoods*. New York: Community Development Research Center Graduate School of Management and Urban Policy New School for Social Research.

Vidal, A. C. (1992). *Rebuilding communities: a national study of urban community development corporations*. New York: Community Development Research Center, Graduate School of Management and Urban Professions. New School for Social Research.

Vidal, A. C. (1989). *Community economic development assessment: A national study or urban community development corporations–preliminary findings*. New York: Community Development Research Center, Graduate School of Management and Urban Professions, New School for Social Research.

Woliver, L. R. (1993). *From outrage to action: The politics of grass-roots dissent*. Urbana, IL: University of Illinois Press.

Conceptual Framework of Coalitions in an Organizational Context

Maria Roberts-DeGennaro, PhD

SUMMARY. Organizations are forming coalitions in their struggle to survive with fewer resources. Under the "Contract With America," funds for human services are expected to be increasingly cut back. Organizational actors will continue to coalesce because of their compelling interests to serve disadvantaged populations in our communities. This article uses the political-economy perspective in presenting a conceptual framework of coalitions in organizational settings. We need access to various perspectives and models of coalition building in order to provide direction for organizational groups as they attempt to change the sociopolitical structures in which they must operate. *[Article copies available for a fee from The Haworth Document Delivery Service: 1-800-342-9678. E-mail address: getinfo@haworth.com]*

KEYWORDS. Coalitions, political-economy, organizational groups, interorganizational collaboration, organizational behavior, coalition building

Human service organizations are struggling to survive with fewer resources. Because of the increased competition for funds, some

---

Maria Roberts-DeGennaro is Professor of Social Work at San Diego State University.

Address correspondence to: Maria Roberts-DeGennaro, Professor, School of Social Work, San Diego State University, San Diego, CA 92182.

[Haworth co-indexing entry note]: "Conceptual Framework of Coalitions in an Organizational Context." Roberts-DeGennaro, Maria. Co-published simultaneously in *Journal of Community Practice* (The Haworth Press, Inc.) Vol. 4, No. 1, 1997, pp. 91-107; and: *Community Practice: Models in Action* (ed: Marie Weil) The Haworth Press, Inc., 1997, pp. 91-107. Single or multiple copies of this article are available for a fee from The Haworth Document Delivery Service [1-800-342-9678, 9:00 a.m. - 5:00 p.m. (EST). E-mail address: getinfo@haworth.com].

91

organizations have agreed to work together in their struggle for survival by forming coalitions. These coalitions provide a convening mechanism through which a group of organizations can interact and work together around a common purpose (Roberts-DeGennaro, 1986a, 1986b, 1987, 1988). Under the "Contract With America," funds for human services are expected to be increasingly cut back due to changes in public policies. In sharing the same compelling interests to serve disadvantaged populations, it is anticipated that these organizational groups will continue to join forces and coalesce.

The author defines a coalition as an interacting group of organizational actors who (a) agree to pursue a common goal, (b) coordinate their resources in attempting to achieve this goal, and (c) adopt a common strategy in pursuing this goal. Stevenson, Pearce, and Porter (1985) defined a coalition as: "an interacting group of individuals, deliberately constructed, independent of the formal structure, lacking its own internal formal structure, consisting of mutually perceived membership, issue oriented, focused on a goal or goals external to the coalition, and requiring concerted member action" (p. 261). For earlier definitions of coalitions, see Gamson (1961), Kelley (1968), Browne (1973), Hill (1973), Van Velzen (1973), and Boissevain (1974).

There are three major advantages for an organization to join a coalition. First, political and economic events are shaking up boundaries, structures, and assumptions related to the delivery of health and human services. In this cost-cutting environment, human service organizations are becoming increasingly motivated to coordinate their efforts and cooperate. As the need for scarce resources intensifies from further funding reductions, organizations are more likely to build coalitions in order to gain or re-gain resources. As a group of organizational actors, a coalition can exert more power and influence and mobilize more resources than a single organization.

Second, as organizational actors interact within a coalition, they are introduced to new ideas, new perspectives, and new technologies for solving problems. This helps to promote an awareness of alternative strategies that the member organizations can use in other problem situations. This interactional process strengthens the coalition's capacity to engage in cooperative problem solving. A sense of empowerment emerges as skills are sharpened in making decisions that people can agree on and enact together.

Third, a more extensive channel of internal communication can be created within the member organizations, as a result of joining a coalition. Representatives from various programs within these organizations may be serving on committees or task forces of the coalition. This involvement serves as a source of feedback to other staff within the organization regarding the coalition's decisions and activities. This feedback loop can help to increase the staff's perspective of how problems affecting their organization also affect other organizations in the community. A "bigger" picture of the problem can then be perceived by the staff rather than maintaining a "lonely organization" perspective.

A review of the literature suggests there is a relative shortage of accepted methodologies for identifying and measuring coalitions. Typically, coalitions have been examined in three- or four-person groups (Stanton & Morris, 1987). Cobb (1991) contends that empirical studies of coalitions have produced a number of important findings, but ". . . the studies were not designed to be generally applicable to coalitions in the organization context" (p. 1058).

The purpose of this article is to present a conceptual framework of coalitions in organizational settings. The objective of the framework is to provide a conceptual context for understanding the diversity of the roles played by coalitions in changing the sociopolitical structures in which they must operate. In developing this framework, first, the political-economy perspective is used to define the nature of coalition building. This perspective represents a broad approach or strategy direction. It suggests that the human services system in which coalitions operate reflects the political processes among those groups that have control over scarce resources, namely, money and authority, and around access to these resources, as well as their allocation (Benson, 1975; Roberts, 1983; Roberts-DeGennaro, 1988).

Next, models of coalitions are used in developing this framework. Models are more specific, detailed, and coherently patterned internally than a perspective, which as previously mentioned, represents a broad approach or strategy direction (Rothman & Tropman, 1987). The author elaborates on Croan and Lees's (1979) five coalition models. In each of these models, the purpose of the coalition dictates the functions to be performed by the coalition. The author then presents case vignettes of these coalition models in order to illustrate their application to practice.

The final section of the article presents some practice considerations in building coalitions. In response to changes in the political-economic environment, coalitions are acting as a convening mechanism for sociopolitical action (Rosenthal & Mizrahi, 1994). For example, instead of waiting for federal health care reform, health care providers are joining forces and creating coalitions to reform the system on their own (Caudron, 1993). In building coalitions, Hagen and Davis (1992) believe there ". . . must be a willingness to compromise so a unified agenda and strategy can be established" (p. 500). As changes in the environment affect the availability of resources, it is suspected that those coalitions which survive will be those that are able to anticipate and adapt to these changes.

Besides using a "survival of the fittest" approach to understanding the behavior of coalitions, we need access to various perspectives and models, in order to develop theories about the practice of coalition building. In the search for a practice theory, this article aims to contribute to the knowledge base related to understanding the diverse roles that coalitions play in adapting to their political-economic environment and in shaping public policies.

POLITICAL-ECONOMY PERSPECTIVE

According to exchange theory, coalitions form in response to the needs of their members as they seek resources from the environment (Levine & White, 1961). Organizations are then driven by resource scarcity to enter into exchanges with other organizations and so they voluntarily form coalitions. Hall, Clark, Giordano, Johnson and Van Roekel's (1977) study supported the contention that when the basis of interaction is voluntary, exchange theory can explain some aspects of a coalition's behavior.

Gillespi and Mileti (1979) argued that resource scarcity is a necessary, but not a sufficient condition for cooperative behavior among organizations in building a coalition. An organization that lacks resources for attaining a particular goal could avert the problem by designating a new goal. Therefore, exchange theory probably cannot predict when an organization might change its goals rather than interact with other organizations and join a coalition.

Benson (1975) extended the basic exchange theoretical framework. He argued, on the basis of Yuchtman and Seashore's (1967) model of acquisition of resources, that organizations seek an adequate supply of money and authority to fulfill program requirements, maintain domain, ensure their flow of resources, and extend or defend their way of doing things. Thus, scarce resources are acquired from a political-economy environment. Due to the nature of this environment, organizations can maximize their supply of money and authority by coalescing with other organizations.

The political environment, within which a coalition operates and performs, refers to the structure of authority and power, and the dominant values, goals, and ethos institutionalized within the coalition. Wamsley and Zald (1973) suggest the coalition carries out political functions in order to insure its growth and survival in this environment, including: (a) defining the mission, ethos, and priorities of the coalition; (b) developing boundary spanning units and positions to sense and adapt to environmental pressures and changes; (c) insuring the recruitment and socialization of the coalition's membership to maintain coherence and the pursuit of the coalition's goals; and (d) overseeing the internal economy and harmonizing it with shifts in goal priorities. These political functions are performed often within a rather turbulent external environment of human service cutbacks and re-organization and/or re-engineering efforts. Consequently, coalitions are continually seeking new elements of community support or potential support for human services and, in some cases, redefining tasks. As a result, they are reshaping the conditions of existence for human services. As change agents, they must know how to generate issues, mobilize constituents, and gain the support of key actors who are affected by and interested in influencing policy.

It is anticipated that political-economic forces will continue to place organizations into competitive positions with other organizations for scare resources. Who has the power in our communities to set the terms of this competition? Usually, it is the local politicians who are elected to represent the needs of citizens in their community. Coalitions are spending a considerable amount of time in preparing documentation for these politicians to demonstrate the needs of disadvantaged clients in order to justify why they need community support.

In preparing documentation on client needs, organizations are expected to develop indicators of performance and establish criteria for effectiveness. In responding to these pressures, information is needed on the outcomes of program efforts and on expected outcomes from future activities. In some coalitions, a core group of members might have the ability to provide technical assistance to other members regarding changes in the requirements for managing programs and reporting program outcomes. Members learn from each other and gain information that is useful to the organizations they represent and that can enhance services to clients (Schopler, 1994, p. 24).

In response to changes in the political-economic environment, coalitions can act as convening mechanisms for community action. Mannix and White (1992) suggest that when coalitions have been operating for a long period of time, they may be the only viable way to get anything done in some political situations. As changes in the environment affect the availability of resources, the coalitions that survive will more than likely be those that are able to anticipate and adapt to these changes.

MODELS OF COALITIONS

In developing a conceptual framework for coalition building, a system of postulates is needed to describe ideal-types of coalitions. This system can then provide a structural design for building coalitions that implies the best possible exemplification either in reality or in conception. Croan and Lees's (1979) five coalition models are used in developing this framework: (a) information and resource-sharing; (b) technical assistance; (c) self-regulating; (d) planning and coordination of services; and (e) advocacy. These models represent a systematic arrangement of categorizing coalitions according to a purpose and a set of functions, which can be performed by the coalition. In each of these models, the purpose of the coalition dictates the type of functions to be performed by the coalition. Table 1 depicts the purpose and functions served by these models.

In "real world" coalitions, one will find some overlap in these coalition models. A coalition may be characteristic of one or more of these models. In the first three models, the coalition works internally to improve the capacities of its member organizations. The last two models attempt to impact externally other systems rather than just their own members.

TABLE 1. Coalition Models

Model	Purpose	Functions
Information and Resource-Sharing	Act as clearinghouse	Gather, collect, file and disseminate information; arrange forums; develop resource-sharing system; assist referral process.
Technical Assistance	Deliver technical services	Arrange workshops; provide grantsmanship and training services; conduct needs assessment and evaluations.
Self-Regulating	Set standards	Design evaluation systems; monitor members; provide certification; recommend system for allocating funds.
Planning and Coordination of Services	Act as service coordinator	Conduct service inventory; establish master calendar; liaise with other groups; develop I & R system.
Advocacy	Act as change agent	Monitor legislation and policy-making bodies; organize public education workshops or campaigns; conduct lobbying efforts.

Note. Preparation of this table was based on material from *Building Effective Coalitions: Some Planning Considerations* by G. Croan and J. Lees, 1979, Arlington, VA: Westinghouse National Issues Center.

The political-economy perspective suggests there are political and economic aspects to understanding the roles played by these coalition models. Zald's (1970) analysis of the political-economy perspective defines these two aspects: (a) the political aspect suggests that organizations within a coalition have various alliances with and commitments to the other member organizations that limit and shape goals, as well as policy choices, and (b) the economic aspect suggests that the member organizations exchange goods, services, or incentives that bind the organizations to each other in the coalition.

Likewise, in each of these models, the alliances and commitments that are developed within the coalition shape the purpose and functions performed by the coalition. In addition, the exchange of goods or services within the coalition creates a bond between the member organizations, which strengthens their interest in maintaining the coalition. Through coalescing, the members anticipate that they will acquire the scarce resources needed by their respective organization.

To illustrate these models, the author has developed case vignettes. It should be noted that the case vignettes are partly fictitious and partly based on actual coalitions. These vignettes are not intended to serve as case studies of these coalition models, but are presented only to briefly sketch the purpose and function of these models.

Information and Resource-Sharing Coalition

According to Croan and Lees (1979), this model serves a definite clearinghouse function. It gathers, collates, files, and disseminates information in specific areas of interest to the coalition. The alliances within the coalition enable the member organizations to achieve objectives such as: (a) providing a means and a forum for exchanging information; (b) developing a knowledge base for organizing and planning activities; (c) providing a system for using the physical facilities, staff, and/or financial resources of the member organizations; and (d) assisting the member organizations in making appropriate referrals.

An information and resource-sharing coalition could publish a newsletter which provides information about special services and events. The coalition can pool available funds in order to purchase, for example, audiovisual equipment or word processing services, that could be used by organizations in the coalition. In some cases, agency staff with special expertise may be loaned or exchanged between the member organizations. Physical facilities such as meeting rooms could be shared. Informal get-togethers can be scheduled in order to nurture the informal network within the coalition. The exchange of these goods and services binds the member organizations to each other as they seek to maximize their scarce resources.

Case Illustration: The Women's Coalition

This coalition was formed in response to a need expressed by numerous women's organizations to bring together the many diverse groups in a state. The common goal of these women's organizations is to collectively influence and lobby for legislation affecting women's rights and economic status. The coalition provides political information, such as action alerts on bills affecting women, in order to strengthen their local lobbying networks. Information is also provided to assist in the appointment of women from the coalition to local and state government boards and commissions.

The coalition publicizes the contributions made by these women's organizations in lobbying for proposed legislation or for changing existing laws that affect the rights of women. Coalition meetings are held throughout the state in an effort to promote communication among the various women's organizations. The coalition is successful in building the capacity of these organizations to respond to women's issues by assisting them to become more informed and knowledgeable in the political arena.

Technical Assistance Coalition

Croan and Lees (1979) suggest this coalition model emphasizes the delivery of technical services. The alliances within the coalition enable the member organizations to receive trainings, conduct evaluations and needs assessments, and arrange other activities on a resource sharing or fee-for-service basis. This coalition model usually operates out of a central office with a coordinator who arranges for the technical assistance. An inventory of the resources, skills, and expertise available within the coalition is often conducted. Outside consultants could be hired, if additional expertise is needed in accessing the technical services.

A technical assistance coalition rarely exists only for improving the service or operating capacity of the member organizations. The technical assistance provided to the member organizations should enable them to affect other systems rather than just their own members. The opportunity to access these services through the coalition creates a bond between the member organizations to each other.

Case Illustration: The Developmental Disabilities Coalition

This coalition is made up of consumer advocate organizations in a state. It sponsors public forums and legislative training workshops across the state, in order to build the capacity of local and state leaders to represent the best interests of the developmentally disabled. Forums consisting of federal, state, or local leaders are coordinated for public hearing purposes. At these forums, disabled persons or their families present testimonies on the major problems and needs of the disabled population in the state.

In conjunction with these forums, legislative training workshops are coordinated for both the disabled citizens and groups working with this population. Experts provide information on the legislative process, in order to assist these groups in learning the "ins and outs" of the political system. The trainers inform the groups on how to organize effective education and communication networks to affect public policy and the decision-making process on behalf of the disabled. Through these workshops, the groups receive information and learn techniques for intervening in this process.

Self-Regulating Coalition

Croan and Lees (1979) suggest this type of coalition assumes responsibility for setting minimum standards by which all the organizations in the coalition agree to abide. Alliances within the coalition enable the member organizations to engage in activities that shape policies. The coalition might design an evaluation system and provide certification for those member organizations that demonstrate compliance. The coalition could monitor its own organizations or even outside groups. It could also recommend to a funding agency a system for allocating funds to its member organizations.

In addition, this coalition model could encourage the upgrading of agency programs and increase standards of performance. For instance, a coalition could be formed by an association of day care centers or a network of emergency shelters to improve their standing operating procedures. Coalescing around these self-regulating activities binds the member organizations to each other. The self-regulating coalition could be formed in combination with the information and resource sharing and/or the technical assistance coalition.

Case Illustration: Youth Shelters Coalition

This coalition consists of several youth emergency shelters in a large metropolitan city. These shelters provide temporary housing and information and referral services for runaway youth. The shelters formed this coalition in response to criticism from local juvenile officials regarding the need to monitor shelter care services. The coalition developed a system for monitoring each of the shelters with the assistance of professional groups interested in children.

Each of the shelters receives monies from the city and the county, as well as local foundations. Representatives from the coalition are asked to recommend to these funding sources the distribution pattern for allocating funds to the shelters. If a shelter is out of compliance with the standards set by the coalition, the shelter can be black-balled by the coalition. As a result, it might not receive a recommendation from the coalition for monies until it is in compliance with the standards. Local funding sources favor the efforts of this coalition, since it provides a watchdog for ensuring quality of care to children in the community.

Planning and Coordination of Services Coalition

According to Croan and Lees (1979), this type of coalition strives to change a situation. The alliances within the coalition provide an avenue for the member organizations to shape goals and policy choices. In order to plan and coordinate services, inventories of existing services, gaps, and duplication of services are often conducted. Other activities might include establishing a master calendar of events, developing a standard intake and referral process, or acting as a liaison with outside agencies. In some cases, experimental or pilot projects might be conducted, which, if successful, could be replicated by other organizations in the coalition.

The formation of this coalition model could be mandated by a major funding source, as a condition in order for the member organizations to receive funds. In this case, a lead organization needs to be responsible for the disbursement of funds, as well as for implementation of the overall project. Participation in the planning and service coordination activities binds the organizations to each other, as they engage in a shared decision-making process to shape goals and policy choices.

Case Illustration: Coalition to Prevent Child Abuse

This coalition was formed by local community-based organizations providing services to victims of child abuse. Member organizations might include parent education groups, private family and youth services organizations, the public child protective services agency, and emergency shelters for battered and neglected children. The coalition conducts an annual resource inventory so that organizations are kept up-to-date on all local resources. A grant proposal is prepared by the coalition for a community development project that would create self-help activities within the community to prevent child abuse.

The coalition makes recommendations to funding sources regarding the fiscal needs of the organizations serving this population. Even though the coalition is not mandated by the funding sources, its recommendations might be used in the allocation of fiscal resources. Therefore, the coalition acts as a liaison between the member organizations and the funding sources.

Advocacy Coalition

Croan and Lees (1979) suggest advocacy coalitions can be formed in response to a specific crisis situation. The alliances within the coalition enable the member organizations to work toward responding to a proposed policy or legislative change, or a more generalized need, such as the lack of home health services. This coalition can also be formed to work towards improving the power base of the organizations in the coalition. Lobbying efforts can be conducted for increasing funding allocations for health and social services, for inclusion of a community representative on a public policy-making board, or for a more equitable distribution of funds.

Organizational actors in an advocacy coalition often serve as members of policy-making boards and monitor legislation or policy decisions. They can organize public education workshops or campaigns to gain support for specific issues, such as a workshop to educate the community on the proposed allocation of federal block grant funds. Their community education work can increase public attention to an issue by the use of various forms of the mass media. This public attention can put pressure on elected decision-makers to be more responsive to the needs of their constituents. Through coalescing around these advocacy efforts, a bond is created between the member organizations, as they seek to maximize their supply of scarce resources.

Case Illustration: Community Coalition

This coalition was formed by a group of alternative human service organizations that were interested in pooling their efforts toward improving their power base. The coalition provides leadership in the community to persuade local government officials to allocate more funds for human services. The leadership puts pressure on local government officials to allocate funds for those human services that might suffer from the loss of funds from federal block grant legislation.

The coalition analyzes local county and city budgets in order to determine if a fair share of the funds are allocated to community-based human services. It advocates for the best use of local monies for human services when the government either contracts out for services or provides its own services. The best interests of the community are continually focused on as the coalition mobilizes its advocacy activities.

PRACTICE CONSIDERATIONS

Regardless of the role played by a coalition in its political-economic environment, Tefft (1987) suggests a coalition faces critical challenges in at least three areas including (a) strategic effectiveness, (b) organizational maintenance, and (c) leadership. A coalition's decentralized structure can limit its strategic effectiveness if decisions are delayed in order to achieve consensus. Decision-making can also become more difficult if member interests are perceived to be jeopardized. If decisions become more controversial within a coalition or go beyond broad issues of values and strategies, the coalition may need to change its structure, including its purpose and functions.

Coalitions often rely on members to maintain the coalition, particularly if there are no paid staff. As member organizations turn over, new organizational actors might not share the same commitment to the coalition. A major challenge would be to identify incentives that will solidify their ideological commitments and integrate them into their working relationships with other members of the coalition. Incentives also need to be provided to the older organizational actors in the coalition in order to enhance their commitment. An organizing ideology needs to promote the spirit of connectedness and solidarity among members (Fisher, 1995).

Stable capable leadership is essential for a coalition's long-term effectiveness. Leadership transition is a predictable, repeated test of a coalition's viability and sense of commitment. The transition from a founding leader or leaders to whatever follows is a critical event. Frequent, unplanned leadership transitions can reduce a coalition's external orientation because of internal demands. The leadership should facilitate the process for the members to agree to some extent on the coalition's purpose, functions, and strategies (Mizrahi & Rosenthal, 1995).

Alexander (1991) suggests one of the first questions to answer in building a coalition is: "What are the precipitating problems or issues that suggest the need for a coalition?" (p. 91). The answer to this question can guide the organizational actors in determining which coalition model or combination of models would best fit their needs.

Daley and Wong (1994) believe practice models of coalition building are needed for working with emerging ethnic communities or between emerging ethnic communities and groups with similar interests. Rivera and Erlich (1984) suggest that these models should nurture and support existing social networks. Gentry (1987) states that in building coalitions an emphasis "should be on cooperation or collaboration between and among agency/organization members and not on competition" (p. 49).

Rather than attempt to establish a grand theory, the intent of this article was to present a conceptual framework that included a perspective or approach to understanding coalition building, as well as a set of ideal types or models of coalitions. Political and economic forces, structures, pressures, and constraints are the most significant motivators of change and the key factors shaping the direction of change for health and human services. Thus, the political-economy perspective should contribute to our understanding of organizational behavior in building coalitions.

REFERENCES

Alexander, C. (1991). Creating and using coalitions. In R. Edwards & J. Yankey (Eds.), *Skills for effective human services management* (pp. 90-102). Washington, DC: NASW Press.

Benson, J. (1975). The interorganizational network as a political economy. *Administrative Science Quarterly, 20*, 229-249.

Boissevain, J. (1974). *Friend of friends: Networks, manipulators, and coalitions.* New York: St. Martin's Press.

Browne, E. (1973). *Coalition theories: A logical and empirical critique.* Beverly Hills, CA: Sage Publications.

Caudron, S. (1993). Teaming up to cut health-care costs. *Personnel Journal, 72*, 104-118.

Cobb, A. (1991). Toward the study of organizational coalitions: Participant concerns and activities in a simulated organizational setting. *Human Relations, 44* (10), 1057-1079.

Croan, G. & Lees, J. (1979, May). *Building effective coalitions: Some planning considerations.* Prepared for the Office of Juvenile Justice and Delinquency Prevention, Law Enforcement Assistance Administration, U.S. Department of Justice. Arlington, VA: Westinghouse National Issues Center.

Daley, J. & Wong, P. (1994). Community development with emerging ethnic communities. In A. Faulkner, M. Roberts-DeGennaro & M. Weil (Eds.), *Diversity and development in community practice* (pp. 9-24). New York: The Haworth Press, Inc.

Fisher, R. (1995). Social action community organization: Proliferation, persistence, roots, and prospects. In J. Rothman, J. Erlich & J. Tropman (Eds.), *Strategies of community intervention* (pp. 327-340). Itasca, IL: F.E. Peacock Publishers.

Gamson, W. (1961). A theory of coalition formation. *American Sociological Review, 26,* 373-382.

Gentry, M. (1987). Coalition formation and processes. *Social Work with Groups, 10*(3), 39-54.

Gillespi, D. & Mileti, D. (1979). *Technostructures and interorganizational relations.* Lexington, MA: Lexington Books.

Hagen, J. & Davis, L. (1992). Working with women: Building a policy and practice agenda. *Social Work, 37*(6), 495-502.

Hall, R., Clark, J., Giodano, P., Johnson, P. & Van Roekel, M. (1977). Patterns of interorganizational relationships. *Administrative Science Quarterly, 22,* 457-474.

Hill, P. (1973). *A theory of political coalitions in simple and policy making situations.* Beverly Hills, CA: Sage Publications.

Kelley, E.W. (1968). Techniques of studying coalition formation. *Midwest Journal of Political Sciences, 12,* 62-84.

Levine, S. & White, P. (1961). Exchange as a conceptual framework for the study of interorganizational relationships. *Administrative Science Quarterly, 5,* 583-601.

Mannix, E. & White, S. (1992). The impact of distributive uncertainty on coalition formation in organizations. *Organizational Behavior and Human Decision Processes, 51*(2), 198-219.

Mizrahi, T. & Rosenthal, B. (1995). Managing dynamic tensions. In J. Tropman, J. Erlich & J. Rothman (Eds.), *Tactics and techniques of community intervention* (pp. 143-148). Itasca, IL: F.E. Peacock Publishers.

Rivera, F. & Erlich, J. (1984). An assessment framework for organizing in emerging minority communities. In F. Cox, J. Erlich, J. Rothman, & J. Tropman (Eds.), *Tactics and techniques of community practice* (pp. 98-108). Itasca, IL: F.E. Peacock Publishers.

Roberts, M. (1983). Political advocacy: An alternative strategy of administrative practice. *Social Development Issues, 7,* 22-31.

Roberts-DeGennaro, M. (1986a). Building coalitions for political advocacy efforts in the human services. *Social Work, 31,* 308-311.

Roberts-DeGennaro, M. (1986b). Factors contributing to coalition maintenance. *Journal of Sociology and Social Welfare, 13,* 248-264.

Roberts-DeGennaro, M. (1987). Patterns of exchange relationships in building a coalition. *Administration in Social Work, 11,* 59-67.

Roberts-DeGennaro, M. (1988). A study of youth services networks from a political-economy perspective. *Journal of Social Service Research, 11,* 67-73.

Rosenthal, B. & Mizrahi, T. (1994). *How to create and maintain interorganizational collaborations and coalitions.* New York: Education Center for Community Organizing at Hunter College School of Social Work.

Rothman, J. & Tropman, J. (1987). Models of community organization and macro practice perspectives: Their mixing and phasing. In F. Cox, J. Erlich, J. Rothman & J. Tropman (Eds.), *Strategies of Community Organization* (pp. 3-26). Itasca, IL: F.E. Peacock Publishers.

Schopler, J. (1994). Interorganizational groups in human services: Environmental and interpersonal relationships. *Journal of Community Practice, 1*(3), 7-27.

Stanton, W. & Morris, M. (1987). The identification of coalitions in small groups using multidimensional scaling: A methodology. *Small Group Behavior, 18*, 126-137.

Stevenson, W., Pearce, J. & Porter, L. (1985). The concept of coalition in organization theory and research. *Academy of Management Review, 10*, 256-268.

Tefft, B. (1987). Advocacy coalitions as a vehicle for mental health system reform. In E. Bennett (Ed.), *Social intervention: Theory and practice* (pp.155-185). New York: Edwin Mellen Press.

Van Velzen, T. (1973). Coalitions and network analysis. In J. Boissevain & J. Mitchell (Eds.), *Network analysis: Studies in human interaction* (pp. 119-225). Netherlands: Mouton and Company.

Wamsley, G. & Zald, M. (1973). The political economy of public organizations. *Public Administration Review, 33*, 62-73.

Yuchtman, E. & Seashore, S. (1967). A system resource approach to organizational effectiveness. *American Sociological Review, 32*, 891-903.

Zald, M. (1970). *Organizational change: The political economy of the Y.M.C.A.* IL: University of Chicago.

Leadership:
Realizing Concepts
Through Creative Process

Si Kahn, PhD

SUMMARY. The paper presents a brief history, context, and theory for community organizing, and provides discussion of major concepts of culture, community, and power. It concludes with a presentation of an interactive training process to tap into the creativity of participants. It illustrates a leadership development exercise that confirms experience and provides affirmation and inspiration for continued organizing work. The process validates participatory leadership, verbally and visually illustrates strengths of participants, and liberates energy for the work. *[Article copies available for a fee from The Haworth Document Delivery Service: 1-800-342-9678. E-mail address: getinfo@haworth.com]*

KEYWORDS. Leadership development, community organizing, social change

Si Kahn is Executive Director of Grassroots Leadership, Charlotte, NC.

Address correspondence to: Si Kahn, Grassroots Leadership, P. O. Box 36006, Charlotte, NC 28236.

This article is excerpted from the author's dissertation, "Standing at the Crossroads: Cultural Work, Community Organizing and Power," submitted to the Graduate School of the Union Institute in 1994.

[Haworth co-indexing entry note]: "Leadership: Realizing Concepts Through Creative Process." Kahn, Si. Co-published simultaneously in *Journal of Community Practice* (The Haworth Press, Inc.) Vol. 4, No. 1, 1997, pp. 109-136; and: *Community Practice: Models in Action* (ed: Marie Weil) The Haworth Press, Inc., 1997, pp. 109-136. Single or multiple copies of this article are available for a fee from The Haworth Document Delivery Service [1-800-342-9678, 9:00 a.m. - 5:00 p.m. (EST). E-mail address: getinfo@haworth.com].

109

INTRODUCTION:
FROM SMALL GROUPS TO LARGE CHALLENGES

One of the many interesting problems in organizing goes something like this: Through the organizing process, people are supposed to become empowered. Because knowledge is power (and because lack of knowledge is in and of itself disempowering), people also need to become knowledgeable. They need new information and new interpretations of old information, along with the tools to acquire and interpret information in the future. But they need to learn all this in ways that are in themselves empowering. If the content of what they learn is contradicted by the way(s) in which they learn it, the organizing and empowerment process undercuts itself and fails.

This, of course, is not just an issue in organizing, but one of the central questions in education broadly and in political education specifically. We know from a variety of contemporary educational theories and practices that people (some would say adults, although these principles really apply to education at any age) learn best when they participate in, shape, define, control their own education (Bastain et al., 1985; Freire, 1972). Participation = empowerment.

This article deals with facilitating participation using a particular small group activity. It provides a theoretical and historical context for community organizing, outlines social change methods, and notes tensions related to professionals and constituencies. Complex issues that organizers deal with ranging from race, gender, and class to power and culture and racial tensions related to autonomous organizations and coalition development are highlighted. The article concludes with an illustration of a group exercise that I developed and have used with grassroots groups and in training groups. The exercise reveals the poetry, passion, and commitment that is expressed when people are asked to complete the phrase: "I am a leader because . . . " Responses in groups to create a poem, a story, and collective wisdom can help to build group culture and bind groups together. Through this exercise, participants move to feeling and creative levels in themselves that can galvanize energy and create a renewed sense of mission that they can bring back to their work tasks. Only one example of this cre-

ative group process is presented here; however, each time that I have used it, the resulting poem has been powerful–conveying meaning and commitment to the possibilities of community organizing. The exercise is one type of small group technique that can be used to build group connections and culture. It operates to confirm leadership and raise collective consciousness about groups and the origins of leadership capacities.

One of the areas where both organizing and education have made substantial progress over the past 30 or so years is in the use of small group techniques. Much of this is due to the influence of the women's movement on organizing and social change work in general (Albrech & Brewer, 1990). The women's movement's development of "consciousness-raising groups" as both an educational and a political technique has been of use and benefit to a wide variety of movements.

I believe one of the reasons that small group consciousness-raising techniques work so well is that they're deeply based on a number of traditional cultural forms, particularly storytelling. As organizers, activists and educators worked with small groups, they discovered that many cultural forms could be adapted to teaching and training. Poetry, written individually and collectively; role-playing; theatre, including "readers' theatre," where parts are read rather than memorized; drawing; painting; singing and songwriting—all of these could, within the framework of the small group, play an effective role. Their importance came partly from the fact that each of these traditional cultural forms, used as a teaching and learning device within the framework of the small group, involved active participation both by individuals and by the group as a whole. People were not the passive recipients of teaching ("banking education," as Paolo Freire named it); they were active and aggressive learners, taking control over their own education and training, and empowered by the process (Freire, 1977).

All this made small group learning very organic, in the sense of "you are what you eat." The method reinforced rather than contradicted the message of empowerment and self-sufficiency. Being part of such groups was rewarding, challenging, exciting, empowering, transforming (Evans, S., 1979).

But at the same time as organizers and activists were learning to use the small group effectively, they were also struggling with the problems of scale (Flacks, 1984). If small is beautiful, it's also often true that large is powerful. In settings where hundreds of people had to be brought together, the small group techniques that had been so carefully developed and polished for the most part didn't apply. To some extent, at conferences and conventions, one could break the large group down into smaller groups, which by definition were equipped to make use of small group techniques. But for those times when the large group met as a whole, and when information needed to be communicated, the only readily apparent solution was to have people sit still and be spoken to, either by individuals or by panels of individuals. While there were and are some great orators among political activists who can bring such a crowd to its feet, that's not the majority of public speakers. Moreover, for many people the act of being spoken *to*, however well, is distancing and disempowering.

After years of being an organizer at the grassroots level, where most of my work was with people in small groups, I began to occasionally be asked to speak to larger gatherings. This worried me for all the reasons outlined above. But was there, I wondered, a way to take the lessons of small group work and apply them to public speaking in a larger gathering? I knew from my experience in the world of music that many performers were experimenting with including other cultural forms in their concerts: storytelling, poetry, call-and-response, dance, theatre.

Could you, I wondered, apply the same principles to public speaking? Within the framework of a public speech, could you draw on and incorporate other traditional cultural forms and techniques, in ways that gave the audience space to participate, at least at an emotional level, and in the process become empowered?

My goal in this story is to document a creative process. In this case (and case study), the process is the one I went through to answer the question which I just posed, by creating and developing a form for public presentation which I've come to call the "song-speech."

One of the turning points that was critical to this process was rediscovering the poetic nature, the rhythm, of much public speech. As with many of my insights that deal with performing (which is to say, with the development of a more or less deliberate public persona and presence), this has developed slowly over a long time. Moreover, this was not a conscious strategy at any point that I recall. Rather, what I'm presenting here in storytelling form is an analysis with hindsight, my own observations on the process I went through over many years to reach this set of conclusions.

CONTEXT I: COMMUNITY ORGANIZING THEORY

Community organizing is a way of life developed and used in all cultures, societies and nations to redress the classic imbalance between the powerless and the powerful. In every known society, contemporary and historical, power and wealth are concentrated in the hands of a relatively few individuals and families. Powerlessness, by contrast, is always in an ironic sense democratically apportioned, a condition shared to some degree by the vast majority of humankind–although, given the operating realities of race, gender and class, by some far more than by others.

Given this universal dynamic, community organizing relies on the power of numbers, of many people thinking, working and acting together, to counterbalance wealth and the multiple means that wealth has to protect, defend, and extend itself: constitutions, governments, bureaucracies, police forces, tax collectors, armies, corporations, caste and class systems, religious institutions, gendered and racialized violence, ownership and control of resources, educational establishments, and communications systems. Whatever the specific issue around which communities organize, the implicit demand is democratization, the redistribution of resources from the few to the many, including both wealth and power.

So community organizing, however carefully it may be publicly described as part of a search for acceptability, respectability, or simple safety and security, is intrinsically radical. It is a call, a cry, a demand for fundamental change, for reapportioning, for restructuring. It is by nature and inalienably a critique of, a set of demands upon, a confrontation with existing economic and political establishments.

From the point of view of any establishment, therefore, community organizing represents a set of potential problems. Whether this dynamic is viewed a mild inconvenience or as a potential revolution depends in part on the balance of power between the forces of community organizing and those of that establishment, whether governmental or corporate.

Establishments that tend towards the authoritarian, whose long-term power is always at risk, work aggressively to restrict community organizing (Fanon, 1968; Memmi, 1967). Their intellectual justifications range from "law and order" to "management rights"; their techniques from anti-union media campaigns to arresting or murdering their own citizens for assembling in groups of more than two or, in some cases, for even speaking to another person without official permission.

Establishments that tend towards the democratic have a more complex intellectual relationship to community organizing. Democratic ideology presumes and advocates not just the consent of the governed but their informed and active participation in that consent. Such consent, to be truthful and effective, must also be collective. That is, in order for any particular constituency to give its informed consent to being governed, whether in the community or in the workplace, it must previously be organized. To deny the right to organize is also to deny the basis on which democratic regimes claim authority, that is, the right to govern (Boyte, 1989).

Democratic establishments therefore tend to deal with the phenomenon of community organizing at least initially by recognizing and institutionalizing it. The constitution of the United States, to take just one example, specifically states in Amendment I of the Bill of Rights that "Congress shall make no law respecting . . . the right of the people peaceably to assemble, and to petition the Government for a redress of grievances." Such language in democratic constitutions provides a legal basis and protection for collective action, that is, for community organizing. Such protections may or may not be reflected in the ongoing realities and dynamics of power and politics.

HISTORY

Within the United States, the development of community organizing can be seen as a response to the multiple forces that combined to create American society, with all of its strengths and weaknesses. Democratic theory, authoritarian institutions, great wealth, dire poverty, personal freedom, chattel slavery, open elections, disenfranchisement of all but property-owning white males, isolationism, imperialism, pacifism, militarism, communitarianism, capitalism, town meetings and political machines are only some among the many complexities and contradictions that shaped this particular civil society.

The United States, then, can be seen as a renewed society drawing on the intersection of many cultures, including particularly in its early phases Native American, African and European. The evolving order embodied in the Declaration of Independence and the Constitution, for example, is indebted to the political theory of the Iroquois Confederation as well as to emerging European ideas of emancipation and communalism. Certainly the New England town meeting, at least in its early form, owes more to the traditions of tribal councils than to those of European councils of state. African cultural and political traditions underpin and inform the development of resistance to chattel slavery by the slaves themselves (Harding, 1981).

All of these ideas find expression in early community organizing efforts. The years leading up to the American Revolution, and particularly the work of the Committees of Correspondence, can be treated as a classic study in community organizing methodology, including recruitment, communication, direct action, coalition-building, fundraising, cultural empowerment and public relations (Boyte, 1989). The Underground Railroad is a remarkable study in how those who are most oppressed can organize themselves, develop both private and public allies, create secure systems of internal communication, develop leadership with the capacity to take risks and hold it accountable (Harding, 1981). Abolitionism depended on a remarkable national network of women who circulated petitions and mobilized their local communities into the movement (Lerner, 1979). Other 19th-century movements such as suffrage, populism, anarchism, craft unionism and pacifism further developed and refined these techniques, including their relationship to issues of race, gender and class.

These 19th-century community organizing movements all have

their 20th-century equivalents and parallels, practitioners and theo-reticians, although these links are often little known or misunder-stood. For example, Saul Alinsky is often claimed as the founder of community organizing, particularly and understandably by members of the Industrial Areas Foundation (IAF), which he founded to continue his work (Alinsky, 1946, 1969). Alinsky's own back-ground, however, draws far more both on social work, especially the work of Jane Addams and Hull House, and on earlier commu-nity and union organizing efforts than this claim would suggest: as a criminology student at the University of Chicago, as a youth worker with Chicago gang members, as the biographer of industrial union leader John L. Lewis. He is an important codifier of and creative contributor to the tradition of community organizing, but hardly the inventor of it (Fink, 1982).

Similarly, other key social movements of our time, which are often thought of as singular and unique, are in fact rooted in and shaped by their own historic ancestors. The civil rights movement of the 1960s owes a great deal to Rosa Parks, Dr. Martin Luther King, Jr., and Malcolm X, but also to Nat Turner, Denmark Vesey, Harriet Tubman, Sojourner Truth, Frederick Douglass, Marcus Garvey, and W.E.B. Dubois (Harding, 1981; Morris, 1984).

As with Addams and Alinsky, the relationship and parallels between the development of community organizing movements and the development of social work are often overlooked. It is too easy to see Hull House and the other founding settlement houses as a type of late 19th-century community development corporation or multi-purpose neighborhood center. The settlement houses were, however, far more radical and far more committed to community organizing than some of their surface resemblances to today's government-sponsored community service centers would suggest. No less a person than Jane Addams herself, the founder of social work as a profession, was a radical, a feminist, a trade unionist, a pacifist, a socialist, an agitator and an organizer (Evans, S., 1989). It is interesting to speculate as to how many social work agencies today would be willing to hire her to direct their social change programs.

SOCIAL CHANGE METHODS

Community organizing is, of course, only one of a number of well-established methods for encouraging and promoting social change. Any analysis of social change strategies depends on a understanding of at least four of these methods: service, advocacy, mobilizing and organizing (Kahn, 1991).

Service attempts to provide people with the basics they need to survive, subsist, develop, and even flourish within society. It is essentially an individualized and personalized approach to social change, which rarely challenges the root causes of the issues addressed. As such, service can address a problem in the short run, but can not solve it in the long run.

A soup kitchen, for example, is a service approach to the problem of hunger. It can insure that, on a given day, a certain number of people are fed. But it cannot and does not address the question of why these people are hungry in the first place. If the soup kitchen folds up, the people it serves will go back to being hungry.

Most of the publicly-supported programs that address social issues take a service approach. Food stamps, job training, public housing, literacy, public assistance, counseling, therapy are all service programs. In a society in which many people do without the basics of life, service programs at their best offer humane relief for suffering. But they are at core helping individuals adjust as best they can to the immediate realities of society, rather than demanding that society change to meet the needs of its individual and collective members. Individuals may be fed, clothed, housed, but they are not empowered. In a certain sense, while service programs may not go as far as directly blaming the victim, they do begin with the assumption that it is the victim that needs to be fixed, not society.

Advocacy begins with the assumption that, if a society includes large numbers of individuals who are suffering, there must be something wrong not just with those individuals but with society as well, and that therefore society as well as individuals must be changed. Concerned citizens who lobby either individually or collectively through their organizations for legislative or administrative changes in programs that affect poor people are practicing advocacy. Legal action to challenge unjust laws and administrative practices are another common advocacy method.

Advocacy does begin to demand changes in society that will benefit its members and, in so doing, begins to raise issues of power and policy. However, in advocacy, these issues are usually raised *on behalf of* those who are affected by the policies and practices in question, but not *by those* who are affected. Advocates, however effective, are representing someone else, not themselves. Thus advocacy can change relationships of power within society, but, because it does not involve people acting on their own behalf, it does not simultaneously empower the disempowered.

Mobilizing begins the process of empowerment by asking people to stand up for themselves. When people show up at a city council meeting to protest the closing of a neighborhood AIDS clinic, when they pass petitions around, when they picket in front of the clinic, when they hold a press conference to denounce the mayor, they are mobilizing. In this process, people who have been disempowered and dispossessed begin to find their voices, to discover confidence, and to feel that they actually have a chance of changing the conditions of their lives and communities.

Because mobilizing is usually a direct response to an immediate situation, it is also limited in what it can accomplish. Sometimes mobilizing leads to such success (or to such frustration) that those involved decide to extend the process and go on to build a community organization. But far more often mobilizing is limited to the immediate situation—and therefore is also limited in both time and scope. It does challenge and sometimes change relations of power, but usually in the short run only.

Organizing as a social change process creates and sustains an ongoing challenge to relationships of power within society (Kahn, 1994). Unlike mobilizing, which takes place within a relatively short time frame, and therefore is unequipped to deal with systemic and structural issues, organizing aims at the building of permanent community organizations that can address and advance the needs of their members. These community organizations then come to constitute a safe space and a separate base of power for those they comprise and represent. Within this space, people who have been disempowered and dispossessed can begin to practice the democratic skills of citizenship and leadership. Through this process they become empowered not just individually but collectively (Evans & Boyte, 1986). They are then able to mount a consistent challenge to the power of established institutions within society.

Such a theory and practice, of course, is far more popular with those who lack power than with those who already have power. Organizing implies a radical critique (which can come from a number of political points of view, from right to left as the spectrum is generally understood) of those in power and of the institutions that they control, including government at all levels (Fink, 1983). Such a critique is rarely encouraged or welcomed by those in power. As a result, they tend to use their position and power to discourage organizing as a social change method, in favor of service or, at worst from their point of view, advocacy.

SOCIAL CHANGE PROFESSIONALS

It should come as no surprise that most institutions and individuals who exercise real power are less than enthused about a philosophy of social change which, from their point of view, can be summarized as "biting the hand that feeds you." This dynamic creates many levels of tension for good-hearted individuals such as teachers and social workers who are, on the one hand, deeply aware of society's inequities and, on the other, heavily dependent on public employment and funding for their own well-being. A social worker may believe that an independent community organization of public housing tenants is the best hope for improving conditions in a particular housing project. But if that same social worker is employed by the public housing authority, they are not exactly in a position openly to encourage and assist that organizing process.

This is a consistent stress to many public and private agency employees with an interest in community organizing. On the one hand, they recognize the systemic causes of the problems they deal with on an individual basis every day, and would like to see structural change take place. They understand and believe that community organizing offers the best hope for such structural change. They may have organizing skill and knowledge themselves: some teachers and social workers did organizing before they enrolled in professional school, others took community organizing courses as part of their professional education. They would like to be able to put this knowledge and skill to good use.

On the other hand, these same public employees are dependent for their own jobs on publicly-funded agencies and institutions which are themselves targets of community organizing efforts. This creates a double bind. To the extent that they identify and work with people who are organizing for power, they run the risk of being monitored, mistrusted, restricted and even disciplined by their employing agency. To the extent to which they are seen as representatives of the agency, they may be monitored and mistrusted by the people they are trying to help. This is a psychologically as well as politically difficult position to be in.

Part of this difficulty comes from the extent to which successful programs developed through independent community organizing efforts are eventually institutionalized and bureaucratized by the public and private sector. For example, in the United States, a major governmental response to the civil rights movement of the 1960s was the "War on Poverty." The local "community action agencies" established across the nation adopted the civil rights movements' emphasis on "participatory democracy" and called for "maximum feasible participation" of the poor. This theoretically admirable principle turned out in practice (at least after congressional action in 1969) that the poor could not ever have *more* than one third of the seats on the governing bodies of these agencies, with two thirds of the seats reserved for those in power. Sadly and ironically, many of the poor people who held these seats and who were hired by these agencies as "community organizers" believed that what they were doing was real community organizing–at least until the point when they attempted to challenge community power, when all too often they found themselves not only powerless but unemployed.

While the "community action agency" case is specific to the late 1960s and early 1970s, the same principle operates broadly today. Individuals and institutions who hold power attempt to undercut and conservatize community organizing by incorporating it in ongoing public programs and agencies. Many people who hold the job title of "community organizer" are in fact limited by agency regulations to service work.

This not only frustrates these individuals; it misleads people in the community at large about the nature of community organizing. The base for community organizing can only exist *outside* the established institutions of society, whether public or private. Because the purpose of community organizations is to change the relationships of power within society, they cannot themselves operate from within the power structure. People do occasionally bite the hand that feeds them, but hardly anyone ever bites their own hand.

CONSTITUENCIES

While community organizing is inherently radical, the techniques and processes known generically as "organizing" are themselves essentially neutral and value-free. The powerful as well as the powerless organize; in fact, effective organizing by the former group is one of the reasons there is such a disparity in power and wealth in so many societies. Right-wingers and fascists as well as progressives and populists adopt and adapt the processes and techniques of organizing to their various ends (Haile, 1979). Organizing can be an authoritarian as well as a democratic technique; organizations can be constructed from the top down as well as from the bottom up.

The particular phrase "community organizing," however, as opposed to simply "organizing," has usually but not always been reserved for when a relatively powerless constituency uses democratic means, including building from the bottom up, to achieve progressive ends. What goals people are working towards, how they are doing that work, and who they themselves are as a group of individuals are therefore critical questions to a definition and exploration of community organizing (Boyte, 1984).

In the language of community organizing, "who people are" is the constituency question. Constituency can be defined by issue (people working towards a particular shared goal or goals); community (people living and/or working in a particular place); and/or identity (people sharing race, class, gender, sexual orientation, religion, ethnicity, age, physical ability, language, tribe). These may of course overlap and intersect: people living in a neighborhood often share a racial and/or ethnic identity and a common set of issues, which may be the result of both where they live and who they are, as well as of both inclusion and exclusion.

One particular community, the workplace, is often excluded from discussions of constituency. "That's labor organizing, not community organizing" is a common statement. This response is ironic, since for many people the workplace is not only where they spend the greatest part of their public time but, given the degree of alienation and rootlessness in modern industrial societies, one of their few consistent communities. This peculiar exclusion reflects both class bias and the degree to which unions threaten the power of modern industrial establishments. Union organizing, however, is as much community organizing as, say, neighborhood organizing. Particularly when it takes gender and race into account, it is critical to a broad and interdependent approach to social change in any culture, society or nation (Brecher, 1972; Fantasia, 1988).

RACE, GENDER, CLASS

Constituency as identity is often defined by race, gender and/or class. Race, gender and class can be thought of as three "lenses," three different but interacting ways of looking at the world and how it works. Viewing the world through any particular lens produces different theories and practices of social change. Looking at the world through the lens of race produces, for example, African national liberation movements and the Southern civil rights movement as practice and Black nationalism and "negritude" as theory. Looking at the world through the lens of gender produces the international women's movement as practice and feminism as theory. Looking at the world through the lens of class produces the trade union movement and multi-national corporations as practice and different economic-based theories of change as theory, including both capitalism and Marxism.

While activists and theorists have argued for centuries as to which of these three forces is the most important, the central factor in determining which position a person takes is usually who they are: a person of color, a woman, a worker. Of course, many people fit into not just one but two or three of these categories: a Native woman, a working class woman, an Asian working class woman

(Davis, 1983). When two or three of these categories are involved at the same time, it's often hard to figure out how they're combining: did she lose the job because she is a woman, because she is an African American—or both?

What is important to community organizing is not to tell people how they should feel about themselves, but to accept their way of looking at the world and to help them build power based on their own analysis. This means that race, gender, and class are not just issues of identity. They are also political forces, rooted in who people believe they are, but affecting also who they believe they could and should be and become (Minnich, 1990). Such dreaming produces powerful momentum, especially when people's identity and sense of themselves has been denied and suppressed both individually and collectively by racism, sexism and/or classism. This sense of personal and collective possibility—who people come to believe through the process of community organizing that they could and *should* be, not just as individuals but as a group, as an organization, as a movement—is one of the phenomena that makes radical and profound social change possible.

SEPARATIST/AUTONOMOUS COMMUNITY ORGANIZING

In the process of organizing around questions of both power and identity, people often want and need to get off by themselves long enough to figure out what they want and how they're going to get it—as well as who they are and how they can take pride in that identity. People who have been exploited and oppressed often need to build a separate base of power for themselves before they can confront their opposition, the people and systems that are the cause of their problems (Evans & Boyte, 1986). Because their base of power is developed separately in this way, this type of community organizing is called "separatism." It's also sometimes referred to as "single-constituency" or "autonomous" organizing. What is important is to recognize separatism not just as a social phenomenon— people wanting to be with others like them—but as a strategic technique for building power.

Many classic forms of community organizing are based on a separatist strategy. Separatism based on class explains why workers don't want management sitting in on the union meeting or joining the union. Separatism based on race explains why people of color may want to join organizations that don't include white people. Separatism based on gender explains why women sometimes want to build organizations that men can't belong to. Of course, since people may have two or three identities these "separatist" categories can also be combined. So, within a local or national union, we might find many "caucuses" (a form of separatist community organizing within a larger community organization): one caucus for Latinas and Latinos, one caucus for women and one caucus for Latinas. Further, one caucus could be related to and make demands on another caucus as well as to and on the larger organization. So the women's caucus might have within it a separate Latina caucus, whose goal was to make sure that in the process of advocating within the union for women the particular needs of Latinas were taken into account.

COALITIONS

While separatist community organizing can be critically important as a social change process, over the long run, many people and organizations that began with separatism will also begin to see a need to work together across the lines that divide them, including but not limited to race, gender and class. One reason for this development is that, in many cases, critical issues cross these and other dividing lines–but are not always seen that way initially by the people whose lives these issues affect.

Toxic wastes are a good example of this phenomenon. When toxic wastes affect the people working in a factory, it's considered a "workplace health and safety issue." When these same toxic wastes are trucked to a poor or working class community and dumped into a leaking landfill, it's described as a "neighborhood issue" or, if the residents of the neighborhood are mostly people of color, as a "racial issue." When children start getting sick from the toxic wastes, it's a "women and children's issue" or a "health issue." When the toxic waste seeps into the nearby streams and fish start dying, it becomes an "environmental issue."

Yet through it all, although the name of the issue may change, the heart of the issue is the same barrel of poison that never should have been there in the first place. The people are different, the communities are different, the issue is named differently. But it's the same fight, with the potential to unite people across lines that would usually divide them.

It's also important to remember that, while some issues are common across race, gender, and class lines, other issues are very different and often in conflict with each other, even between and among so-called "progressive" community organizations (Bulkin, Pratt & Smith, 1984; Evans, S., 1979). For example, there is a real conflict between established systems of seniority, a principle central to working class organizations (trade unions), and affirmative action, a principle equally central to organizations of women and/or people of color. For community organizers to pretend that these differences and conflicts don't exist, that "It's all the same struggle," that "We're all in this together" in the same way is asking one party or the other to give up something that is central to its organization, issue and identity. In both the short and the long run, this is asking for trouble.

However, it's also true that those who are in power ordinarily oppose both affirmative action and seniority. With remarkable consistency, those who are against the rights of people of color also oppose the rights of women and the rights of working people. There are some exceptions, such as a few labor and/or civil rights supporters who are against reproductive rights. But generally, an important reason to build organizations that cross race, gender, and class lines is that, even where the issues really are different, two things are the same: the opposition and a broad vision of a different and better world.

People and communities may not always agree on what's the most important issue to work on at a particular time. But they can often agree that the ways in which power is exercised and by whom need to be changed before they or anyone else can win on their issues. If there is one great issue that can unite across race, gender, and class lines, it is power: who has it and who doesn't, how it can be transferred and transformed by a positive and affirming vision of a world in which people and communities are valued and respected because of, not in spite of, who they are and can be (Kaye/Kantrowitz, 1992).

MOVEMENTS AND ORGANIZATIONS

In the language of community organizing there's a saying that "organizers organize organizations." This is not just a definition but a prescription. That is, it's generally considered practical and reasonable for a community organizer or a team of community organizers to set out to decide to build a new organization from the ground up (Kahn, 1994). If their analysis of conditions was reasonably accurate, if their strategy and tactics are sound, if they do their job conscientiously and well, then that organization will most probably be built.

But community organizers are only rarely able to organize movements, those periods of rapid and profound transformation which are essential to an ongoing process of social change. Movements occur only when certain economic, political and social conditions are right for that movement to happen (Bloom, 1987). Even the most skilled community organizers can't ordinarily succeed in deliberately organizing movements, although many have tried. In fact, it's even hard to see movements coming very far in advance. Very few people predicted the great anti-colonial movements in Africa beginning in the 1950s, the civil rights movement in the southern United States during the 1960s or the international women's movements of the 1970s.

On the other hand, it seems safe to say that major social change movements do and will occur with some regularity, and that therefore the coming decades will see many such movements throughout the world. Once these movements are under way, their possibilities of success will have a lot to do with the skills and abilities people involved in any particular movement have on hand. It will depend on how clearly they can see what to do, with how good their "ize" are: their abilities to mobilize, organize, strategize, publicize.

The movement will also be influenced by the degree to which people have learned and not learned to understand, work with and trust each other. So whenever and however the next movement starts in the world, its future will very much depend on the leaders, organizers, organizations, networks, and coalitions that community organizers have helped develop during the prior non-movement years. Therefore, in non-movement periods, community organizers must work to create the conditions and resources that will make a movement most effective once it begins to happen.

As any movement reaches its peak and begins to ebb, it needs to find ways to consolidate and protect the gains it has won. The new leadership that had emerged and developed in the course of the movement needs to find outlets for its energy, creativity, and commitment. One of the ways all this happens is through the building of community organizations that can out-last the waning of the movement, can carry on its work, and can provide the space within which newly-emerged leaders can continue to grow. Thus within a period of movement, the work of community organizers is to continue organizing, to institutionalize and formalize, to build and sustain organizations that can carry on the work and power of the movement after it ebbs. This process is also accompanied by realignments of power and wealth, and can result in everything from new neighborhood organizations to new governments.

POWER AND CULTURE

Community organizing, however, must change more than power. It must also change the relationship that the people being organized have to power. This means that community organizing must work to change *how people think about and relate to themselves and others* (Minnich, 1990).

In the language of community organizing, this is the political education question. It addresses what is often a weakness of community organizing, that it can become (in ways typical of the dominant cultures in today's world) technological, instrumental, linear, manipulative. People and communities may win on the issues, but that doesn't necessarily mean they develop new understandings of how and why they won, of power and how it is exercised, of difference and how it is exploited. They may experience the power of numbers, but not necessarily the concurrent power of knowledge, of understanding. Some of the conditions of their lives may change, but they will not necessarily transform their relationship to others (particularly their relationships to others different from themselves, to "the other"), to themselves, to power itself (Mihnich, 1990).

These transformations lie in the realm and are the responsibility of political education. Yet traditional educational methods, which are fundamentally intellectual, aren't always adequate to deal with a transformative process, particularly one which challenges racism, sexism, homophobia, anti-semitism and other barriers that divide people from each other. Breaking through such barriers requires velocity, momentum, torque, acceleration of the spirit as well as of the mind. It is a visceral and emotional as well as an intellectual process.

Such emotional and visceral breakthroughs are the expertise of culture and "cultural work," the conscious and strategic use of culture, craft and art to achieve political goals. Poems, songs, paintings, murals, chants, sermons, quilts, stories, rhythms, weaves, pots, dances can literally lift people out of themselves–and sometimes even into the life and consciousness of another self, of someone quite different from their self, from themselves. The power of culture can also be an antidote to people's racialized and gendered inertia, to their inability to see beyond their own eyes. If community organizing can transform power, cultural work can transform consciousness, can perform the acts of political education that, combined with community organizing, make social change transformative rather than merely instrumental.

Yet within the world of community organizing, cultural work is too often (to paraphrase Charlotte Bunch's famous quote about women and "history") a matter of "add music and mix." Cultural workers and cultural work itself are often minor adjuncts to the community organizing process: a quilt at an auction, a song or two at a rally, a chant on a picket line. Many community organizers have yet fully to recognize and to incorporate into their daily and working lives and work the lessons of culture and cultural work, to draw on the full power that they can provide. Community organizing needs to draw on and incorporate the full variety of traditional and non-traditional forms from many cultures: oral poetry, storytelling, *midrash*, meditation, quilting, theatre, preaching, drumming, unaccompanied song, silence.

This is the critical challenge to community organizers and social workers today: how do you organize people, how do you reach and teach them, in ways that transform their understanding of power and their relationship to power–not just individually, but collectively, so that not only power but community is built. It is at this intersection of culture and power that the future of community organizing and of social change must be found.

"I AM A LEADER BECAUSE"

For example: in December, 1993, at the Grassroots Leadership Annual Conference, I was assigned to facilitate a workshop on "leadership," with about 20 people present in a small room, about half African Americans and half white people. I wanted the workshop, which was scheduled to last for two hours, to be participatory and to set the leadership themes which concerned the group. Ten years ago I would have asked everyone to take a few minutes to think about and/or write down the ideas on leadership they wanted to discuss. We would then have gone around the room in a circle to the left, always to the left, with each person adding one item to the overall list, which would simultaneously be written down on a newsprint flip chart, until there were no ideas left unsaid. The consolidated list would then have provided the framework for the discussion of leadership which was to follow.

This time, given the thinking I've been doing about culture, community and power, I wanted something more dramatic, powerful and personal. The instructions I gave to the group were:

1. Stand up.
2. Say, "My name is _____ and I am a leader because . . ." and then go on to complete the sentence.
3. Tell us about one "elder" from your family or community who helped you become the leader you are today.

I asked each person to keep their presentation to under two minutes. As there was no flip chart in room, I took verbatim notes as each person spoke. My intention had been to read through the notes continuously as different members of the group spoke in turn, underlining the common themes that occurred so I could present them as a framework for discussion. But as I listened, wrote and read, I became struck with the sheer poetry of what was being said. When the last person finished, I thanked the group and asked if, before beginning the discussion, they'd like to hear a poem about leadership. They said "yes." I told them the name of the poem was "I Am a Leader Because" and I began to read:

I am a leader
because I jump in
I am a leader because I have respect for people—
and for difference
I am a leader because my grandfather wore a red tie
and did exactly as he pleased

I am a leader
because I'm dissatisfied with the current leadership
I am a leader because I'll fall in line with anyone
who's doing a good job
I am a leader because I'm committed
to having my attitudes
attest to my work and struggle for others
I am a leader because there was a need for change in leadership
and a chance for personal growth

I am a leader
because my grandmother was determined
and never recognized failure in herself
I am a leader because
with no father and nine brothers and sisters
I was thrust into that area of responsibility
early in my life
and because my grandmother
who lived to be 113 years old
had a caring, compassionate spirit

I am a leader
because I can empower people
I am a leader because my dad was interested in everybody
I am a leader because I was told as a child
that I was rebellious
and because I had questions
no one could answer

I am a leader
because I am outspoken
committed to excellence and compassion
and because my grandmother doesn't believe
in 'no'

I am a leader
because I like to work with people
to take responsibility–
and because I don't mind taking responsibility
if others do too

I am a leader
because I'm never satisfied with the status quo
and because the nature of life
is to grow and expand
I am a leader because I like challenge
ask questions
and do research
I am a leader because I listen
because I try to craft my ideas
and philosophies
around what I hear
not just what I believe

I am a leader
because I can make things happen
and because I can enable other people's views to happen
I am a leader because I'm a roleplayer
because there's a lot of work
to be done
I am a leader
because there's always people in my neighborhood
who call on me

I am a leader
because I'm a good listener
I am a leader
because I can move people

I am a leader because
you could see the hard times
on his face

I am a leader
because I don't think of myself
as a leader
I am a leader because I'm a facilitator
for other people to be in leadership positions

I am a leader because other people
have encouraged me
to speak about what I know
and want

I am a leader
because I am one of the worker bees
I am a leader
because my name means
'growing and appreciative'

I am a leader
because everybody is a leader
by nature
I am a leader
because there are always people
who are following you

I *might* be a leader
because I *may* have a voice
that some people
are afraid
to use
sometimes

When I finished reading, there was a long moment of silence and
then big grins. Someone said, "We really wrote that, didn't we."
They spent a little time telling each other how good what they had
said was and then we moved on to discussing what they had heard

and to other elements of the workshop. About five minutes before the workshop came to a close, I asked if they'd like to hear the poem again as a final ceremony and, when they said, "yes," read it a final time.

An interesting sidelight: the crew that was videotaping the gathering walked in just after I had started reading the poem for the first time. After the workshop was over, one of the video crew members came up to me and asked who had written the poem and whether they could get a copy of it. I repeated this question to the group who all said proudly, "We did."

I was fascinated by what happened here, more or less accidentally. It was clear that the exercise, intended simply as an icebreaker and to generate some ideas for discussion, had created a powerful sense of community, however temporary, among members of the group. This sense of community had also pushed their personal presentations, questions and analyses in a deeper direction, resulting in a remarkably candid and open discussion of leadership. When we moved into a part of the workshop where people were asked to play roles, some of which involved racial and/or gender shifts, they responded with remarkable skill and lack of inhibition. *Through using this exercise with this group and other groups, I have learned that it becomes a means to build collective culture, open participants to creativity, and renew commitment to organizing projects. The exercise is more than an "exercise to go through," it becomes a powerful learning and affirming experience within the group. It unleashes shared creativity, a much needed and often overlooked critical component of community organizing.*

REFERENCES

Adams, Frank, with Myles Horton, *Unearthing Seeds of Fire: The Idea of Highlander*, John F. Blair, Winston–Salem, 1975.

Albrecht, Lisa and Rose M. Brewer, *Bridges of Power: Women's Multi-Cultural Alliances*, New Society Publishers, Philadelphia, 1990.

Alinsky, Saul D., *Reveille for Radicals*, Vintage Books, New York, 1969.

Alinsky, Saul D., *Rules for Radicals: A Pragmatic Primer for Realistic Radicals*, Random House, New York, 1971.

Barnard, Hollinger F., *Outside the Magic Circle: The Autobiography of Virginia Foster Durr*, Simon and Schuster, New York, 1985.

Bastian, Ann, Norm Fruchter, Marilyn Gittell, Colin Greer and Kenneth Haskins, *Choosing Equality: The Case for Democratic Schools,* New World Foundation, New York, 1985.

Bloom, Jack, *Class, Race and the Civil Rights Movement: The Changing Political Economy of Southern Racism*, University of Indiana Press, Bloomington, 1987.

Bobo, Kim, Jackie Kendall and Steve Max, *Organizing for Social Change: A Manual for Activists in the 1990s*, Seven Locks Press, Cabin John, Maryland, 1991.

Boyte, Harry C., *Commonwealth: A Return to Citizen Politics*, The Free Press, New York, 1989.

Boyte, Harry C., *Community Is Possible: Repairing America's Roots*, Harper and Row, New York, 1984.

Boyte, Harry C., *The Backyard Revolution: Understanding the New Citizen Movement*, Temple University Press, Philadelphia, 1980.

Brecher, Jeremy, *Strike!*, Straight Arrow Books, San Francisco, 1972.

Buhle, Paul, *C.L.R. James: The Artist As Revolutionary*, Verso, London, 1988.

Bulkin, Elly, Minnie Bruce Pratt and Barbara Smith, *Yours in Struggle: Three Feminist Perspectives on Anti-semitism and Racism*, Long Haul Press, Brooklyn, 1984.

Carawan, Guy and Carawan, Candie, *Songs for Freedom: The Story of the Civil Rights Movement Through Its Songs*, Sing Out Publications, Bethlehem, Pennsylvania, 1990.

Carson, Clayborne, *In Struggle: SNCC and the Black Awakening of the 1960s*, Harvard University Press, Cambridge, 1981.

Clark, Paul F., *The Miners' Fight for Democracy: Arnold Miller and the Reform of the United Mine Workers*, New York State School of Industrial and Labor Relations/Cornell University, Ithaca, 1981.

Conway, Mimi, *Rise Gonna Rise: A Portrait of Southern Textile Workers*, Anchor Press/Doubleday, Garden City, New York, 1979.

Davis, Angela Y., *Women, Race and Class*, Random House, New York, 1981.

Denselow, Robin, *When the Music's Over: The Story of Political Pop*, Faber and Faber, London, 1989.

Delgado, Gary, *Organizing the Movement: The Roots and Growth of ACORN*, Temple University Press, Philadelphia, 1986.

Dunson, Josh, *Freedom in the Air*, International Publishers, New York, 1965.

Evans, Eli N., *The Lonely Days Were Sundays: Reflections of a Jewish Southerner*, University Press of Mississippi, Jackson, 1993.

Evans, Eli N., *The Provincials: A Personal History of Jews in the South*, Atheneum, New York, 1973.

Evans, Sara M., *Born for Liberty: A History of Women in America*, The Free Press, New York, 1989.

Evans, Sara M., *Personal Politics: The Roots of Women's Liberation in the Civil Rights Movement and the New Left*, Alfred A. Knopf, New York, 1979.

Evans, Sara M. and Harry C. Boyte, *Free Spaces: The Sources of Democratic Change in America*, Harper and Row, New York, 1986.

Fanon, Frantz, *The Wretched of the Earth*, Evergreen Press, New York, 1969.

Fantasia, Rick, *Cultures of Solidarity: Consciousness, Action and Contemporary American Workers*, University of California Press, Berkeley, 1988.

Flacks, Richard, *Making History: The American Left and the American Mind*, Columbia University Press, New York, 1989.

Foner, Eric, *A Short History of Reconstruction*, Harper and Row, New York, 1990.

Foner, Philip S., Editor, *Mother Jones Speaks: Collected Speeches and Writings*, Monad Press, New York, 1983.

Foner, Philip S., *Organized Labor and the Black Worker 1619–1973*, There International Press, New York, 1976.

Freire, Paulo, *Pedagogy of the Oppressed*, Herder and Herder, New York, 1972.

Garafalo, Reebee, *Rockin' the Boat: Mass Music and Mass Movements*, South End Press, New York, 1988.

Garrow, David J., editor, *The Montgomery Bus Boycott and the Women Who Started It: The Memoir of Jo Ann Gibson Robinson*, University of Tennessee Press, Knoxville, 1987.

Geoghegan, Thomas, *Which Side Are You On? Trying To Be for Labor When It's Flat on Its Back*, Farrar, Straus and Giroux, New York, 1991.

George, Nelson, *The Death of Rhythm and Blues*, Pantheon Books, New York, 1988.

Giddings, Paula, *When and Where I Enter: The Impact of Black Women on Race and Sex in America*, William Morrow and Company, New York, 1984.

Hallie, Philip, *Lest Innocent Blood Be Shed: The Story of the Village of Le Chambon and How Goodness Happened There*, Harper and Row, New York, 1979.

Harding, Vincent, *There Is A River: The Black Struggle for Freedom in America*, Vintage, New York, 1983.

Jones, Bessie, and Bess Lomax Hawes, *Step It Down*, University of Georgia Press, Athens, Georgia, 1987.

Jones, Mary Harris, *The Autobiography of Mother Jones*, Charles H. Kerr Publishing Company, Chicago, 1990.

Kahn, Si, *How People Get Power* (second revised edition), National Association of Social Workers Press, Washington, 1994.

Kahn, Si, *Organizing: A Guide for Grassroots Leaders* (second revised edition), National Association of Social Workers Press, Washington, 1992.

Kaufman, Jonathan, *Broken Alliance: The Turbulent Times Between Blacks and Jews in America*, Charles Scribner's Sons, New York, 1988.

Kaye/Kantrowitz, Melanie, *The Issue Is Power: Essays on Women, Jews, Violence and Resistance*, Aunt Lute Books, San Francisco, 1992.

Kivnick, Helen, *Where Is the Way: Song and Struggle in South Africa*, Viking Penguin, New York, 1990.

Lerner, Gerda, *The Majority Finds Its Past: Placing Women in History*, Oxford University Press, New York, 1979.

Marable, Manning, *Race, Reform and Rebellion: The Second Reconstruction in Black America*, 1945-1982, University Press of Mississippi, Jackson, 1984.

Memmi, Albert, *The Colonizer and the Colonized*, Beacon Press, Boston, 1967.

Minnich, Elizabeth Kamarck, *Transforming Knowledge*, Temple University Press, Philadelphia, 1990.

Mitchell, H.L., *Mean Things Happening in This Land: The Life and Times of H.L. Mitchell, Cofounder of the Southern Tenant Farmers Union*, Rowman, Landham, Maryland, 1979.

Mitchell, H.L., *Roll the Union On: A Pictorial History of the Southern Tenant Farmers' Union*, Charles H. Kerr Publishing Company, Chicago, 1987.

Morris, Aldon D., *The Origins of the Civil Rights Movement: Black Communities Organizing for Change*, The Free Press, New York, 1984.

Nelson, Jack, *Terror in the Night: The Klan's Campaign Against the Jews*, Simon and Schuster, New York, 1993.

Oates, Stephen B., *The Fires of Jubilee: Nat Turner's Fierce Rebellion*, Harper & Row, New York, 1975.

Omi, Michael and Howard Winant, *Racial Formation in the United States: From the 1960s to the 1980s*, Routledge and Kegan Paul, New York, 1986.

Pharr, Suzanne, *Homophobia: A Weapon of Sexism*, Chardon Press, Inverness, California, 1988.

Reagon, Bernice Johnson and Sweet Honey in the Rock, *We Who Believe in Freedom*, Doubleday, New York, 1993.

Rosenberg, Daniel, *New Orleans Dockworkers: Race, Labor and Unionism 1892-1923*, State University of New York Press, Albany, 1988.

Seeger, Pete and Bob Reiser, *Carry It On! A History in Song and Picture of the Working Men and Women of America*, Simon and Schuster, New York, 1985.

Seeger, Pete and Bob Reiser, *Everybody Says Freedom: A History of the Civil Rights Movement in Songs and Pictures*, W.W. Norton and Company, New York, 1989.

Staples, Lee, *Roots to Power: A Manual for Grassroots Organizing*, Praeger, Westport, Connecticut, 1984.

Terkel, Studs, *Race: How Blacks and Whites Think and Feel About the American Obsession*, New Press, New York, 1992.

Ward, Robert D. and William W. Rogers, *Labor Revolt in Alabama: The Great Strike of 1894*, University of Alabama Press, University, Alabama, 1965.

White, Timothy, *Catch A Fire: The Life of Bob Marley*, Henry Holt and Company, New York, 1992.

Woodward, C. Vann, *The Strange Career of Jim Crow* (third revised edition), Oxford, New York, 1974.

Zinn, Howard, *SNCC: The New Abolitionists*, Beacon Press, Boston, 1964.

Index

Note: Page numbers followed by t indicate tables.

Abolitionism, community
    organization in, 115
Addams, J., 33,116
Advocacy
    in community-based development
        model, 71-72
    definition of, 117-118
Advocacy coalition, 97t,102-103
Affordable housing industry, CBDOs
    in, 60
Alexander, C., 104
Alinsky, S., 20,33,116
American Revolution, community
    organization in, 115
Autonomy, in community
    organization, 123-124

Banks, CBDOs and, relationships
    between, 73-74
Believing in change, 22-23
Benson, J., 95
Bower, B., 18,22,23
Bunch, C., 128
Business skills, teaching of, by
    CBDOs, 69-70

CARECEN (Central American
    Refugee Center), 36,38t
CBDOs. *See* Community-based
    development organizations
Center for Community Change, 77
Central American Refugee Center
    (CARECEN), 36,38t,43-44
Checkoway, B., 5

Child abuse, prevention of, coalition
    in, 102
Civil rights movement, community
    organization in, 116
Clark, J., 94
Coalition(s)
    advocacy, 97t,102-103
    community, 103
    in community organization,
        124-125
    in community-based development
        model, 76-79
    definition of, 92
    developmental disabilities, 100
    identifying and measuring of,
        methods, 93
    information and resource-sharing,
        97t,98-99
    in organizational settings
        advantages of, 92-93
        challenges facing, 104
        commitment to, 104
        conceptual framework of,
            91-107
        decision-making in, 104
        for gaining resources, 92
        indications for, 94
        interactional process in, 92-93
        internal communication in, 93
        leadership of, 104
        models of, 96-103
            advocacy coalition, 97t,
                102-103
            information and resource-
                sharing coalition,
                97t,98-99

137

planning and coordination of
  services coalition,
  97t,101-102
self-regulating coalition, 97t,
  100-101
technical assistance coalition,
  97t,99-100
political environment of,
  description of, 95
political-economy perspective
  in, 93,94-96
questions related to, 104
resource scarcity and, 94
technical assistance for, 96
planning and coordination of
  services, 97t,101-102
practice considerations, 104-105
to prevent child abuse, 102
self-regulating, 97t,100-101
technical assistance, 97t,99-100
women's, 99
youth shelters, 101
Collier, Rev. J., 42
Commitment, of community workers
  and leaders, 8
Committees of Correspondence,
  community organization in,
  115
Communication, internal, through
  coalitions, 93
Community
  definition of, 13
  general welfare of, 14
  as intervention in society, 14
  strengthening of, 13-15
  forms of, 13-14
Community change
  core concepts for, 11-29. *See also*
    Core concepts
  agents of change as, 20-21
  believing in change as, 22-23
  developing leadership as,
    19-20
  empowerment as, 23-25
  focus on people as, 17-19

getting organized as, 16-17
joining together in solidarity,
  15-16
multicultural process, 25-26
strategies, 21-22
strengthening community as,
  13-15
voluntary action as, 20
empowerment in, 23-25
multicultural, 25-26
skills in, 21
strategies in, 21
styles in, 21
support networks in, 20
voluntary action in, 20
Community coalition, 103
Community interventions,
  description of, 14
Community organization
  advocacy in, 117-118
  founder of, 116
  history of, 114-116
  leadership in, 109-136. *See also*
    Leadership, in community
    organizing
  mobilizing in, 118
  models of, Gulfton, 31-34. *See
    also* Gulfton
  organizing in, 118-119
  problems of scale in, 112
  separatist/autonomous, 123-124
  service in, 117
  small group techniques in, 110-113
  social change professionals in,
    119-121
  social work and, 116
  theory of, community organizing,
    113-114
Community organizing theory,
  113-114
Community practice
  CBDOs and, 85-88
  models of, 1-9. *See also*
    Conceptual models for
    community work

Community Practice: Conceptual Models, 4-5
Community Reinvestment Act, 71
Community-based development model, 57-90. *See also* Community-based development organizations
empowered, 65-85
  advocacy in, 71-72
    in development within neighborhoods, 73-76
  Alinsky-style organizer in, 77
  coalitions in, 76-79
    tactics of, 78-79
  funding for, 76
  government's role in, 79
  holistic development of, 65-71
  lease purchase home ownership programs in, 67
  limitations facing, 86
  loan funds for, 66,76
  organic theory in, 80
  social conscience in, 79-85
  social services and physical redevelopment in, 65-71
  support structure in, 76-79
Community-based development organizations (CBDOs), 57-90
  abandoning organizing for development by, 64-65
  academics' views of, 58
  advocacy agenda and, 58
  advocating for development within neighborhoods by, 73-76
  in affordable housing industry, 60
  attitudes and beliefs of, 86
  balance between bottom line and obligation to help people in, 63
  banks' relationships with, 73-74
  business skills training by, 69-70
  community organizing by, 71

definition of, 57
development projects in
  description of, 60
  types of, 60-61
developmental activists' role in, 59
direct actions by, 71-72
domination of neighborhood associations by, 64
double bottom line facing, 61-64
economic development projects stimulated by, 70
homeowners' and tenants' counseling by, 65
hospital saving by, 73
job training by, 65
"keeping projects afloat by," 62
as landlords, trade-offs in, 62-63
lessons for community practice by, 85-88
neighborhood advocacy issue weakening by, 64
neighborhoods of, 62
New Communities Corporation, 68-69
physical development by, 65
progress achieved by, 60
protests against, 73-74
resources for, 61
rules developed by, 67
school building refurbishing by, 74-75
social agencies and, relationship between, 67-69
social obligation *versus* financial wherewithal facing, 62
and social quality, 87
street-level community organizers in, salary of, 75
success of, 60-61
  questions related to, 61-65
types of, 59
wealth to neighborhood through, 70
Community-building, 14
  limitations of, 14-15

Conceptual models for community
  work, 1-9
  adaptability in, 3-4
  application of, 4
  characteristics of, 2-3
  creativity in, 3-4
  definition of, 1
  description of, 1
  evaluation of, 4
  hybrid models, 3
  participants in, creativity of, 8
  types of, 4-5
Constituency(ies)
  in community organization,
    121-122
  definition of, 121
Core concepts
  for community change, 11-29. *See
    also* Community change,
    core concepts for
  description of, 11
  purposes of, 12
  sources of, 12
Counseling
  homeowner, by CBDOs, 65
  tenant, by CBDOs, 65
Crime, in Gulfton, 36
Croan, G., 93-94,96-103
Culture, in community organization,
    127-129

Daley, J., 105
Day-care centers, subsidized,
    trade-offs in, 62
Developmental activists, role in
    CBDOs, 59
Developmental disabilities coalition,
    100
Douglass, F., 116
Dubois, W.E.B., 116
Dudley Street Neighborhood
    Initiative, 64

Education, community organization,
    49-51
Empowerment
  in community change, 23-25
  in community organization
    leadership, 110
Empowerment through ownership, in
    community development,
    79-85
Encyclopedia of Social Work, 4
Erlich, J., 105

Financial accountability, *versus*
    social goals, 62
Fisher, R., 5-6,47
Freire, P., 23

Gamble, D., 4
Garey, M., 116
Gender, as factor in community
    organization leadership,
    122-123
Gentry, M., 105
Getting organized, as core concept in
    community change, 16
Gillespi, D., 94
Giordano, P., 94
Gittell, M., 72
Goetz, E.G., 64-65,71,72,77
Grassroots Leadership Annual
    Conference, 129-132
Gross, S., 72
Gulfton
  apartment complex construction
    in, 34-35
  community organization in, 31-56
    Central American Refugee
      Center, 43-44
    consensus organizing
      strategies in, 33
    description of, 36-46
    diversity of, 46-49
    educational implications in,
      49-51

effects on Shenandoah
  neighborhood, 37,39-40
Gulfton Area Action Council,
  40-42
Gulfton Area Neighborhood
  Organization, 45-46
Gulfton Area Religious
  Council, 42-43
multiple publics in, 34
reasons for, 36
Shenandoah Civic Association,
  36,37,38t,39-40
social work approach to, 47
Southwest Houston Task
  Force, 44-45
crime in, 36
development of, 34-36
economic collapse in, 35
ethnicity and racial breakdown in,
  34
Latino immigrants in, 35
oil industry effects on, 34-35
size of, 34
standard of living in, 36
Gulfton Area Action Council
  (GAAC), 36,38t,40-42
Gulfton Area Neighborhood
  Organization (GANO), 37,
  38t,45-46
Gulfton Area Religious Council, 36,
  38t,42-43
Gutierrez, L.M., 24

Habermas, J., 32
Hall, R., 94
Homeowner counseling, by CBDOs,
  65
Horton, M., 23
Houston, Texas, Gulfton community
  organization in, 31-56. *See
  also* Gulfton, community
  organization in
Hull House, 116
Hyde, C., 3,44

"I Am A Leader Because," 129-132
Immigrants, Latino, in Gulfton, 35
Industrial Areas Foundation, 116
Information and resource-sharing
  coalition, 97t,98-99

Jeffries, A., 1-2,4
Job training, by CBDOs, 65
Johnson, P., 94
Joining together in
  community-building, 15-16

Kahn, S., 7-8
Kaufmann, L.A., 48
Kennedy, E., 44
Kieffer, C., 24
King, Dr. M.L., Jr., 116

Landlords, CBDOs as, trade-offs in,
  62-63
Lanier, Mayor, 39
Latino immigrants, in Gulfton, 35
Leadership
  in coalitions, 104
  in community change,
    development of, 19-20
  in community organizing,
    109-136. *See also under*
    Community organization
  class in, 122-123
  coalitions in, 124-125
  constituencies in, 121-122
  culture and, 127-129
  empowerment in, 110
  gender in, 122-123
  group learning in, 11
  history of, 114-116
  "I Am A Leader Because,"
    129-132
  movements and, 126-127
  power in, 127-129
  public speech and, 112-113

race in, 122-123
small group technique in,
110-113
social change methods, 117-119
social change professionals,
119-121
Lease purchase home ownership
programs, CBDOs and, 67
Lees, J., 93-94,96-103
Lewis, J.L., 116
Local Initiative Support Corporation,
76-77
Lord, S., 44
Low Income Housing Tax Credit, 77

Malcolm X, 116
Mannix, E., 96
Mansbridge, J., 33
Marston, S.A., 35-36
Mileti, D., 94
Movements, organizations and,
126-127
Multiculturalism, in community
change, 25-26

New Communities Corporation, 68-69
Newman, K., 72

Oil industry, effects on community
organization in Gulfton,
34-35
Organic theory, in community
development, 80
Organization(s), coalitions in,
conceptual framework of,
91-107. *See also* Coalition(s),
in organizational settings
Organizing
as core concept in community
change, 16-17
description of, 16-17

Parks, P., 116
Pearce, J., 92
Physical redevelopment, in
community-based
development model, 65-71
Planning and coordination of
services coalition, 97t,
101-102
Popple, K., 2-3,4
Porter, L., 92
Power, in community organization,
127-129
Private life, description of, 33-34
Public life
description of, 32
in Gulfton, 31-56. *See also*
Gulfton, community
organization in
importance of, 50-51
Public speech, in community
organization, 112-113

Race, as factor in community
organization leadership,
122-123
REHAB Network, 77
Rice, P., 42
Rivera, F., 105
Roberts-DeGennaro, M., 7
Rothman, J., 2-3,4,47
Rubin, H.J., 6
Ryan, M., 32

Seashore, S., 95
Self-regulating coalition, 97t,
100-101
Separatism, in community
organization, 123-124
Service(s), definition of, 117
Shenandoah Civic Association, 36,
37,38t,39-40
Sidney, M., 64-65,71,72
Sisters of Charity Southwest Health
Clinic, 44-45

Skill(s), definition of, 21
Social change
  community organizing in,
    117-119
  professionals in, 119-121
Social goals, *versus* financial
    accountability, 62
Social services
  CBDOs and, relationship
    between, 67-69
  in community-based development
    model, 65-71
Social work, community
    organization and, 116
Social work practice, community
    organization education and,
    49-51
Socioeconomic factors, as factor in
    community organization
    leadership, 122-123
Solidarity, in community-building,
    15-16
Southwest Houston Task Force,
    36-37,38t,44-45
Stevenson, W., 92
Stoecker, R., 58
Strategy(ies)
  in community change, 21
  definition of, 21
Style(s), definition of, 21
Sullivan, M., 65
Support networks, in community
    change, 20

Taafe, L., 5-6
Technical assistance coalition, 97t,
    99-100
Tefft, B., 104
Tenant counseling, by CBDOs, 65
Towers, G., 35-36
Truth, S., 116
Tubman, H., 116
Turner, N., 116

Underground Railroad, community
    organization and, 115

Van Roekel, M., 94
Vesey, D., 116
Vidal, A.C., 71
Voluntary action, in community
    change, 20

Wamsley, G., 95
Weil, M., 4
Werner, D., 18,22,23
White, S., 96
Women's coalition, 99
Wong, P., 105

Youth shelters coalition, 101
Yuchtman, E., 95

Zald, M., 95

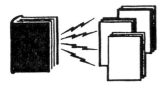

Haworth
DOCUMENT DELIVERY
SERVICE

This valuable service provides a single-article order form for any article from a Haworth journal.

- *Time Saving:* No running around from library to library to find a specific article.
- *Cost Effective:* All costs are kept down to a minimum.
- *Fast Delivery:* Choose from several options, including same-day FAX.
- *No Copyright Hassles:* You will be supplied by the original publisher.
- *Easy Payment:* Choose from several easy payment methods.

Open Accounts Welcome for ...
- Library Interlibrary Loan Departments
- Library Network/Consortia Wishing to Provide Single-Article Services
- Indexing/Abstracting Services with Single Article Provision Services
- Document Provision Brokers and Freelance Information Service Providers

---

MAIL or *FAX* THIS ENTIRE ORDER FORM TO:

Haworth Document Delivery Service
The Haworth Press, Inc.
10 Alice Street
Binghamton, NY 13904-1580

or FAX: 1-800-895-0582
or CALL: 1-800-342-9678
9am-5pm EST

PLEASE SEND ME PHOTOCOPIES OF THE FOLLOWING SINGLE ARTICLES:

1) Journal Title: _____
   Vol/Issue/Year: _____ Starting & Ending Pages: _____
   Article Title: _____
   _____

2) Journal Title: _____
   Vol/Issue/Year: _____ Starting & Ending Pages: _____
   Article Title: _____
   _____

3) Journal Title: _____
   Vol/Issue/Year: _____ Starting & Ending Pages: _____
   Article Title: _____
   _____

4) Journal Title: _____
   Vol/Issue/Year: _____ Starting & Ending Pages: _____
   Article Title: _____
   _____

(See other side for Costs and Payment Information)

COSTS: Please figure your cost to order quality copies of an article.

1. Set-up charge per article: $8.00
   ($8.00 × number of separate articles) _____

2. Photocopying charge for each article:

   1-10 pages: $1.00 _____

   11-19 pages: $3.00 _____

   20-29 pages: $5.00 _____

   30+ pages: $2.00/10 pages _____

3. Flexicover (optional): $2.00/article _____

4. Postage & Handling: US: $1.00 for the first article/
   $.50 each additional article _____

   Federal Express: $25.00 _____

   Outside US: $2.00 for first article/
   $.50 each additional article _____

5. Same-day FAX service: $.35 per page _____

GRAND TOTAL: _____

METHOD OF PAYMENT: (please check one)

❑ Check enclosed ❑ Please ship and bill. PO # _____
(sorry we can ship and bill to bookstores only! All others must pre-pay)

❑ Charge to my credit card: ❑ Visa; ❑ MasterCard; ❑ Discover;
❑ American Express;

Account Number: _____ Expiration date: _____

Signature: ✗ _____

Name: _____ Institution: _____

Address: _____

_____

City: _____ State: _____ Zip: _____

Phone Number: _____ FAX Number: _____

MAIL or *FAX* THIS ENTIRE ORDER FORM TO:

Haworth Document Delivery Service
The Haworth Press, Inc.
10 Alice Street
Binghamton, NY 13904-1580

or FAX: 1-800-895-0582
or CALL: 1-800-342-9678
9am-5pm EST)